Hamilton Bailey

A Surgeon's Life

Hamilton Bailey

A Surgeon's Life

by

Adrian Marston

CAMBRIDGE
UNIVERSITY PRESS

CAMBRIDGE UNIVERSITY PRESS
Cambridge, New York, Melbourne, Madrid, Cape Town, Singapore, São Paulo

Cambridge University Press
The Edinburgh Building, Cambridge CB2 8RU, UK

Published in the United States of America by Cambridge University Press, New York

www.cambridge.org
Information on this title: www.cambridge.org/9780521518819

First published 1999
Digitally reprinted by Cambridge University Press 2008

A catalogue record for this publication is available from the British Library

ISBN-13 978-0-521-51881-9 hardback

THE BACKGROUND TO THE STORY

This is the story of a famous surgeon. Famous surgeons are today an extinct species. Up to the middle of this century, someone who had inherited or learned the manual skills needed for reconstructing the human body, combined with a capacity to command and dominate those around them, was an admired figure. Medical science has now advanced to the point where that sort of person is no longer needed or employable. The glamour has disappeared. Accurate imaging of body processes has made it possible to identify and correct anatomical faults in fellow creatures without having to go through a process that involves first poisoning them and then cutting them open. In developed countries, society will demand that these problems be dealt with by a new sort of professional, who will have been trained to heal broken organs, remove tumours and deal with infection, in fact to do all the things that surgeons used to do, employing virtual technology and visio-spatial skills. Attempts to label this person as a radiologist, surgeon, or technician will be seen as a dispute between artisans, rather than as a reflection of social need. Experts of the new type will supplant the ancient academies and colleges, whose accumulated funds will be used for historic and charitable purposes, much like the old guilds and trades unions. They will be servants of society, rather than guardians of tribal wisdom, and their performance will be managed, scrutinised and priced. Today's skills are tomorow's barbarities, and it is likely that before long surgery will be looked upon as just another ancient craft, and the term 'surgeon' will become as picturesque as 'cobbler' or 'wainwright'.

But things were not always so, and there is one famous surgeon whose name has survived for more than a century, and may even outlast the present revolution. Hamilton Bailey was not particularly dexterous, and his relationship with patients and colleagues was often uneasy. His reputation is preserved through his writings and his ability to communicate to others a vast store of knowledge and experience, so that the books that he wrote have run into scores of editions, still bearing his name. Of all those who have ever written about surgery, Bailey is still by far the most widely read. Furthermore, he had a strong and inspirational character, and led an unusually adventurous life.

This is not the first biography. In 1973 the Ravenscourt Press published S. V. Humphries' short *Life of Hamilton Bailey* which has been an invaluable source of material for the new book, and I acknowledge my debt. Humphries was the sort of surgeon who made an immediate and impressive impact on any one who met him (I never did), but was quite unknown to the general public and indeed to most of his own profession. A slight, modest figure, totally selfless and idealistic, he spent his entire working life in mission hospitals in various parts of Africa, including Malawi, Transvaal and Pondoland, never seeking any sort of publicity or recognition, and on the one occasion at which he was given a minor honour, turned up in tropical kit, having forgotten to hire clothes suitable for the event. Most of the time he worked alone, relying on texts and atlases to guide him through difficult unfamiliar operations, and like most surgeons in similar circumstances, found that by far the most useful books were those written by Hamilton Bailey, with whom he corresponded but never met. Humphries retired to Málaga in 1973, and there worked in close collaboration with Veta Bailey on her husband's 'Life', the only book he ever wrote. Inevitably, there were constraints, and in deference to her and to the memory of the man he so revered, some of the more painful aspects of the story were omitted or at least glossed over. Humphries died in 1982, Veta in 1989, and Bailey has no surviving relations, so that the whole account can now be told for the first time.

I have also drawn on Eric Jewesbury's *History of the Royal Northern Hospital 1856-1956*, although, interestingly, he says nothing about that Hospital's most famous surgeon, beyond listing his name. My other chief source of information was the Bailey papers which I found disintegrating in the basement of the Royal Northern, and also the records of the Royal London Hospital which were made available to me by the kindness of the Archivist, Mr Jonathan Evans. It is good to know that the Bailey collection is now in his capable hands. Additionally, I would like to thank the friends and colleagues who have given much time and thought to contributing information and memories. Sadly, not all of them are still alive. They include:

Surgeons and other colleagues from the RNH:

Hugh Baron, Stephen Carstairs, Allan Clain, Zina Fitzgerald, Tony Green, Alan Kark, Rex Lawrie, Leslie Le Quesne, Reginald Murley, Ian Robin, Albert Singer, Valentine Swain, James Thomson (senior and junior).

Psychiatrists:

Desmond Hanbury, David Rice, Neil Joughin, (Chichester), Guy Goodwin (Oxford).

Co-Authors, Editors and Publishers:

John Lumley, Tony Raines, Paul Remes.

And in addition:

John Farndon (Bristol), Peter Bevan, Ian Donovan, George Hearn (Birmingham), Roger Grace, Patrick Thorn (Wolverhampton), Clifford Brewer, Robert Shields (Liverpool), James Watt, Tony Revell (Royal Navy), Cameron Moffatt (British Red Cross).

D. A. Scales (Ramsgate), Stan Durrant (Bishopstoke), Mrs J. P. Farnell (Preston Central Library), Mrs J. Lambert, Michael Berry, Anthony Poole (Mill Hill).

Charles Beamish, Jill Osborne, San Bon Matsu, Manuel Verdugo, Juan Verdugo (Fuengirola and Mijas).

Finn Hanberg-Sørensen (Aarhus), Robert van Hee (Antwerp).

D. J. Toomey (Gibraltar).

Elisabeth Braam (International College of Surgeons), Alison Stevenson (Royal College of Surgeons of Edinburgh).

About The Author

Adrian Marston trained in Oxford, London and Boston, and worked for many years in the National Health Service as a consultant surgeon to The Middlesex and the Royal Northern Hospitals. He has been Vice-President of the Royal College of Surgeons, and President of the Association of Surgeons of Great Britain and Ireland, and of the Vascular Surgical Society. He is an honorary member of the French and Spanish Surgical Associations and is the author of five surgical textbooks and some 130 papers in scientific journals. Following four years as Dean of the Royal Society of Medicine, he was elected Vice-President in 1998.

Contents

Chapter 1
ANTECEDENTS

Hamilton Bailey's story starts with his father, Dr James Bailey, who was born at Forfar, Scotland in 1864, the son of a mining engineer. He was hard working and able, and to the pride of his parents gained entrance to the Medical School of the University of Edinburgh and qualified as a doctor (MB ChB) in 1887. The indirect accounts we have of young James' character suggest that he was a somewhat dour individual, conscientious, dutiful and not an easy socialiser. Three years after qualifying and following junior appointments in hospitals in Scotland and the South of England, including short periods in Brighton and in the Naval Hospital at Portsmouth, he married Margaret Bailey (no relation) whom he had met as a nurse at the Edinburgh Royal Infirmary, and, together, as dedicated Christians, they joined the Mission field. In 1890, James was appointed as medical superintendent of the Church Missionary Society hospital in Nablus in Palestine, the main town of what is now the West Bank, but which was then part of the Ottoman Empire, and a place that has for centuries been a centre of religious and political conflict. Formerly known as Sckechem, it was the holy city of the Samaritans, and their temple on Mount Gerizim still overlooks the centre. The Samaritans were always a despised minority (hence the Biblical parable of the good one) but in view of their ancient territorial claim that they are the only Jews who have always been around in the homeland, they have now been more or less accepted into Israeli society. We have few details of the Baileys' life in Nablus, but one can imagine the difficulties of a young Scottish couple, attempting to preach the Christian Gospel and practice medicine in a dusty, hostile environment, with few drugs and instruments, and not much to offer over and above the skills of the local practitioners. They spoke no Arabic or Hebrew, and Margaret's situation as a Western female must have been even more constricted than that of a nurse in Saudi Arabia today. They could certainly set fractures and open abscesses, and coming from Edinburgh with its long tradition of obstetrics, they probably delivered babies more skilfully and less destructively than did the local village women. They also had the mixed advantages of being unofficial representatives of British imperial power, with all of the respect, authority and odium which that carried, though the Baileys would probably have preferred to overlook such a connection. They must have felt physically uncomfortable for much of the time, hot, tired and not too well fed, vulnerable to all the bacteria and parasites of the Middle East, with little understanding of hygiene, nor of the elementary principles of rehydration.

Margaret became pregnant very shortly after their arrival in Nablus, but continued to work. It was not surprising that a baby born in those unpropitious conditions died at the age of two days. Later evidence suggests that it was a son. Margaret developed a puerperal illness which seems in the first instance to have been a fever, but was rapidly followed by a full-scale depression, during which she developed the conviction that she had been the direct cause of the baby's death, an idea which would haunt her for the rest of her life. She became silent and withdrawn, with outbursts of uncontrollable weeping. Later accounts suggest that the loss of their child in these difficult circumstances was borne fairly stoically by James Bailey, in contrast with the devastating effect that it had on his young wife. Life in Nablus became hard to bear. Dr Bailey applied to the Church Missionary Society for release from his contract, and the young couple returned to Scotland in the autumn of 1891.

According to her sister Edith, who was 16 at the time of their return, Margaret arrived from Palestine in a highly fraught and unstable condition, quite unable to make any rational decision. James, on the other hand, was calm and determined. He at first searched for work in and around his native Edinburgh, but soon discovered, as had many of his compatriots, that Scotland already had more than enough doctors, so that he looked towards the more affluent South of England. He had already worked in Brighton and Portsmouth, but found no opening there, and his discovery of a vacant practice in the village of Bishopstoke in Hampshire was exactly what was needed. Lying on a bend of the river Itchen between Winchester and Southampton, Bishopstoke provided the sort of rural peace which James was seeking after his harsh experiences in the mission field, and gave him some hope that the environment would provide a haven for his wife to recover her balance. The fact that he was a keen fisherman may have contributed to its appeal. The family found a house ("Hazelmere") in the quiet St Mary's Road, next to the church, settled in and began to establish a practice. But this seemingly tranquil village had been caught up in the wake of the industrial revolution and was in fact the scene of bitter social conflict.

Bishopstoke

Until the mid-nineteenth century, Bishopstoke had been an entirely agricultural community, most of whose inhabitants worked on the land or in related crafts such as thatching, milling, harness-making or in the smithy. Regular paid employment was hard to come by, and families were forced to earn a little extra from such work as grave-digging and stone-breaking. Children from the age of seven were expected to earn their keep, and were hired out to local farmers. The community was poor and undernourished, and deaths were frequent from fever, consumption and dysentery. Those who through old age or infirmity were unable to work were housed in the poorhouse, founded in 1793 and maintained at the expense of the parish until 1840. In that year the character of the village underwent a radical change, with the opening of the London to Southampton railway, which made travel easier, and brought into the village not only workers connected with the railway, but also wealthier families who found in Bishopstoke pleasant rural surroundings within easy reach of the nearby towns. Tension arose between the established farmers and county families, the new arrivals from Southampton and Portsmouth (many of them military or naval officers), and the agricultural workers and railway employees, most of whom came from distant parts of the country or from Ireland, and were resented as foreign invaders. This situation became much worse in 1885 when the London and South Western Railway moved its main depot from Nine Elms in London to Eastleigh, just a mile from Bishopstoke. This provoked a rapid rise in population with the acquisition of farming land for the construction of terraced housing for the new working class. The old church, which had stood on the village green overlooking the river Itchen since 1825, became too small, and a wealthy local man, Mr Alfred Barton, offered a new site together with £1000 towards the building costs, on condition that "all the seats should be free". A bitter dispute flared up between the benefactor and the owners of "faculty pews" in the old church. They had paid for exclusive use of their high-walled box pews, which in the absence of the owners remained empty, so that the ordinary members of the congregation were obliged to stand at the back of the church, once the limited free seating had been taken up. The newcomers were quite unused to these feudal ways, and expressed their resentment loudly and publicly. The argument rumbled on for years, long after the new church was completed in 1891, with the pew owners and established families attempting to preserve the old church, which was rapidly deteriorating. An attempt was made to maintain Divine Service there but the Bishop ruled that this could only be done if the parishioners paid for a curate, and this they were not prepared to do. The local doctors were dragged into the dispute and the District Medical Officer, Dr Harnett, declared the old churchyard unsafe for burials ("considering that the public Elementary Schools are directly opposite..."). We do not know what stand Dr Bailey took on this issue, but it is probable that he sided with the parishioners, in opposition to Dr Harnett. The Winchester Consistory Court was asked to intervene, but the matter was not finally laid to rest until the old church was finally demolished in 1906.

James' son Hamilton was born at Bishopstoke, in their new house in Scotton Road, on 1 October 1894. The birth was uncomplicated, and Edith, who now had started to train as a nurse, came down to help the family out. Margaret must have been comforted by the safe arrival of a healthy little boy, in circumstances so different from those in Nablus, but James was less secure. He remained in

Bishopstoke for two more years, but eventually the pressures occasioned by the unsettled nature of the village, and the uncertain future of a single-handed practice in that environment, drove him to look for alternatives. Other doctors were arriving. The panel system had yet to be introduced, and the older established families, who could afford to pay for medical care, were moving out into the countryside, or into Portsmouth and Southampton, whereas the railway families and agricultural workers were economising on fees.

When a practice vacancy became available further down the river, the decision was easy. In 1896 James and Margaret and their two year old son moved from Bishopstoke to 37 Church Street, Southport, where quite soon another child was born, a daughter named May. May inherited many of the features of her mother. From the first she was a disturbed and troublesome child, who behaved badly in public, and was difficult to know. Later, the parents sought professional help and were told that May was mentally ill, the diagnosis being "dementia praecox", or what would now be called schizophrenia. This illness was a source of shame and embarrassment to the family, and it seems that the little girl was not allowed out of the house. There are no records of her in any of the surviving papers. Hamilton was brought up as if he had been an only son, and in later life he never mentioned his sister. This shadowy aspect of the family life was successfully concealed from the public, because a hint of a scandal of such a nature would have prejudiced the success of Dr Bailey's medical practice. Much later on, at the age of 18, May was consigned to St Francis' Mental Hospital at Haywards Heath (Figure 1.1) where she eventually underwent a prefrontal leucotomy, and from which she never emerged.

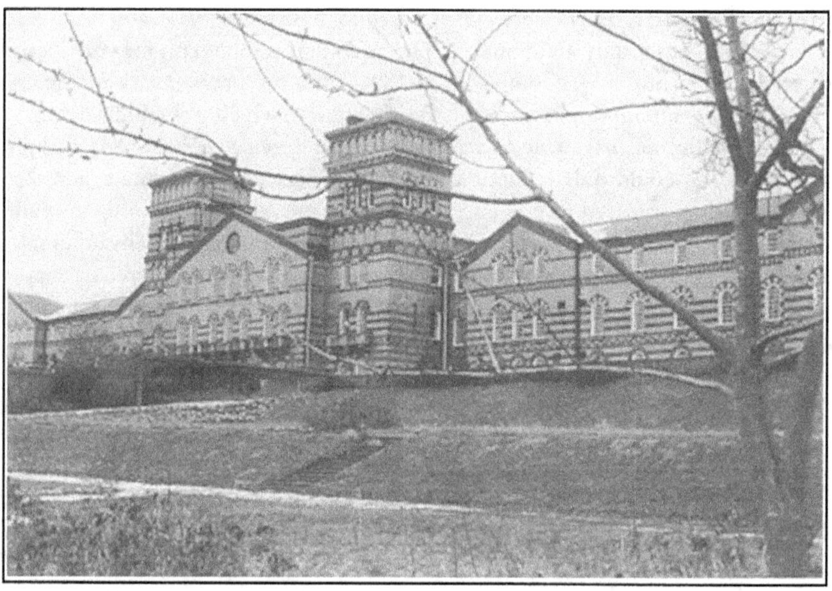

Figure 1.1: St Francis' Hospital, Haywards Heath, formerly the Sussex County Lunatic Asylum

There is little information regarding Dr Bailey's time in Southport, but as no partners are recorded in the Medical Directory, it seems that he must have been in single-handed practice. In any event he spent only two years there, and in 1898 moved to Eastbourne, where he practised from No. 13 Cavendish Place. This again was a temporary stopping place, pending his final move to Brighton, where he had briefly worked as a young doctor and where he was to spend the next 30 years.

Brighton and Hove

At the beginning of the nineteenth century, the former small Sussex fishing village of Brighthelmstone had been transformed by the Prince Regent into a fashionable marine resort. Since then, Brighton had expanded and grown rich, and at the time of the Baileys' arrival it was at its heyday as a prosperous residential and semi-industrial town, with a Royal Pavilion, fine theatres, hotels and restaurants, magnificent Georgian architecture, an aquarium, two piers and flourishing tourism. There were in fact three distinct communities in the Brighton complex. The richest of these centred around the imposing seafront hotels, The Metropole and The Grand (Figure 1.2), where multinational deals were sealed over brandy and cigars, the Old Ship which attracted the local gentry and merchants, and The

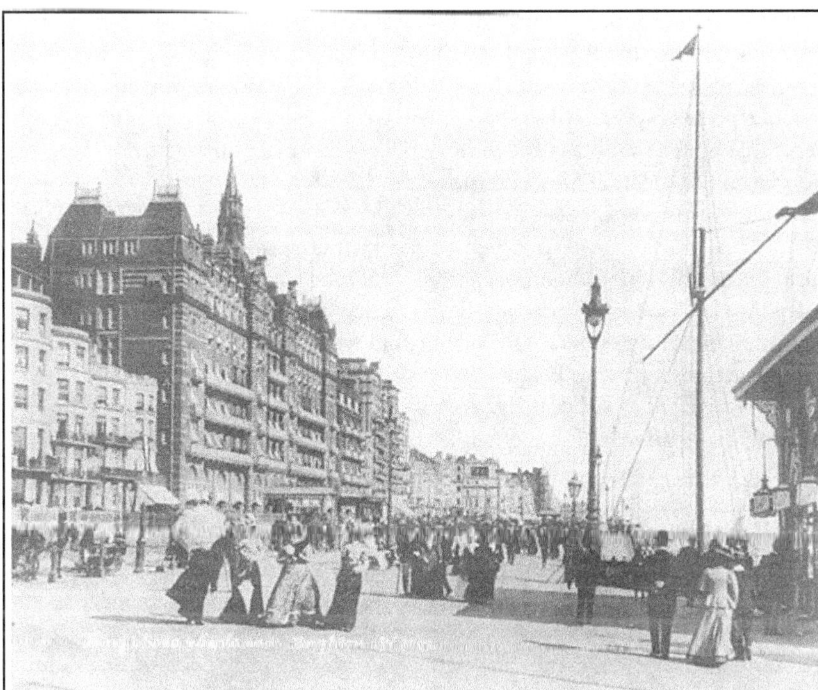

Figure 1.2: The Brighton Seafront 1904, showing The Metropole Hotel in the background (Courtesy of the Brighton Museum).

Norfolk which was much patronised by the Jewish community. Brighton was a major commuter town for senior managers in the City of London, exactly one hour from Victoria Station (time for a hand of whist on the Brighton Belle with its silverware and fringed lampshades), whose homes lay mainly in the Regency squares and the cliffs of Kemp Town and the Marine Drive.

At the opposite end of the social range, Brighton competed with Southend in Essex in providing a day at the seaside for the working people of London with cockles and whelks, a free shingle beach, Volk's model railway, saucy postcards, a racecourse, Louis Tussaud's waxworks, the Albion football club and hundreds of cheap eateries. The communities collided in a somewhat farcical way through the divorce industry, as the easiest way to end a painful marriage was to produce proof of adultery ("two pairs of shoes outside the bedroom door, your Honour") and Brighton with its large number of prostitutes and small hotels was ideally placed to provide the necessary facilities. Parallel with and partly as a result of these social contrasts, there was the large and flourishing criminal underclass, as described by Graham Greene in *Brighton Rock*, centred around the greyhound track and racecourse. But all this mixture of history, vulgarity, crime, money and fun depended on the third Brighton, the people who lived there and ran the place, the building contractors, bank managers, shopkeepers and assistants, small firms of solicitors, secretaries and innumerable servants, who were Dr Bailey's patients, and whose lives young Hamilton saw at close range as he accompanied his father on his rounds. The family home at No. 100 Rugby Road lay in a quiet residential area of the town, inhabited for the most part by this sort of people. A few patients came to the house, but Margaret did not welcome this, and the main practice premises were at No. 88 Lewes Road, a busy commercial street, easily accessible both to shoppers and visitors. The occasional "carriage trade" was important to the success of the enterprise.

This was the town in which young Hamilton grew up, to which he returned from his school holidays, and in which he observed his father's increasingly busy and successful practice. The practice was on the approved list of both Brighton and Hove, so that Dr Bailey could work in either place, and although Hove is continuous with Brighton it was and still is a very different sort of town. On the sea front, the boundary is marked by an inconspicuous mark on the pavement and a winged statue, while the terrace of renaissance mansions overlooking the Channel continues imperturbably across the dividing line (Brunswick Square and Adelaide Crescent are as good as anything Brighton or Kemp Town have to offer). However, inland Hove is quite distinct. Whereas Brighton was a County Borough in its own right, which meant that it had its own local government, Hove lay in the county of West Sussex and was subject to the restraining influences of the rural background. The excitement, the raffish and glamorous criminal elements, the music, the drama and the colour of Brighton were matched in Hove by a degree of respectability which in its sheer stuffiness becomes almost exotic. Hove was a town whose prosperity depended on the elderly, the wealthy and the retired. Every day, scores of Bath chairs could be seen moving slowly along the sea front, the occupants, their knees securely tucked into tartan rugs, propelled by attendants often almost as decrepit as themselves. Crime in Brighton meant muggings and knifings in the street, with motorbikes screaming away into the darkness. Crime in Hove, if ever detected, implied terrible things done behind lace curtains and hidden in the cellar.

To a local doctor, the divide was quite simple. Brighton people by and large were supported by charity or were on the panel. Hove people paid directly. Dr Bailey's dual appointment gave him access to the Brighton, Hove and Preston Dispensary, founded in 1846 where patients without means could receive treatment. The stipend was small, but the professional satisfaction was high. and there were indirect benefits. As the dispensary lay in Hove, it received charitable support from middle-class families, a connection which gave Dr Bailey entry into the more affluent society which supported the private side of his practice.

But there was a problem. Margaret's mental illness, which had started following the death of her first child in Nablus, and had survived two others, recurred in active and vengeful form. She was beautiful, manipulative, very sociable, and unwilling (and probably unable) to take on the responsibilities demanded of a general practitioner's wife. It has been rumoured that she found it hard to resist the approaches of her husband's more influential patients, which would have been in character, but if she was unfaithful to her husband, no proof remains. What is certain is that she was so preoccupied with her personal problems that she could not relate to her growing son and mentally deranged daughter, whom she treated with alternating bouts of affection and abuse. Soon after the family arrived in Brighton, she started to drink heavily. Quite often, Dr Bailey would be summoned from the surgery back to Rugby Road by the Police because his wife had been found insensate in the middle of the town and brought home in a cab. He bore these episodes with a certain stoicism, but the impression develops that, in order to continue his professional life, he felt the need to isolate himself from emotional incursions, which meant that he was unable to express love and affection (always assuming that he felt them) not only to his increasingly alienated wife, but also towards young Hamilton.

Margaret was treated intermittently at a private mental hospital at Ticehurst near Tunbridge Wells in Kent, but Dr Bailey's practice could not support this for long and, as expenses mounted, she was transferred during her periods of instability to an institution at Haywards Heath which had started life as the Sussex County Lunatic Asylum, then became the Brighton Borough Mental Hospital, and was eventually given the decorous name of St Francis Hospital. The buildings still stand as a huge, empty mausoleum in the grounds of new Princess Alexandra Hospital, which now serves the local Sussex community (Figure 1.1). This type of institution typified the enlightened Victorian attitude to mental illness. Instead of the barbarities of Bedlam where madmen were chained in cages for the amusement of the populace, the nineteenth-century philanthropists built palatial asylums for the reception of lunatics, surrounded usually by large gardens tended by the inmates. Gardening was not only therapeutic but also made economic sense, in that any of the produce not consumed on the premises could be sold to help support the asylum. Each county had one or more of these institutions, and the county of London necessarily had a great number, situated outside the centre, where land was cheaper. To the north were Napsbury and Friern, and to the south, Netherne and Banstead. There were similar large asylums to the East and West of the capital, in an area referred to by cynical civil servants as "the loony belt". St Francis in Sussex was absolutely representative of this type of institution. Almost certainly, the rejected daughter May would have been in the hospital at the same as her mother, but the records have disappeared.

Hamilton grew up in a family overshadowed by mental illness, which they tried, not always successsfully, to conceal. There were bouts of angry alienation, where the faults of an adolescent were harshly criticised, and his small successes disregarded. A few years later on, when he timidly informed his mother that he had failed a medical school entry examination, her reply was "you fool!". This small incident is an example of what must have been typical of his family life.

Perhaps luckily for all parties concerned, there was a safety valve for family tensions, which was the uniquely British institution of the boarding Preparatory School (preparatory, that is, for the Common Entrance examination to one of the major Public Schools). Originally created for the needs of temporary orphans of army officers or parents serving in India and other unhealthy parts of the Empire, they soon became the accepted norm for the education of boys of eight to twelve years of age from middle-income families: accepted at least by the fathers but often to the great distress of the small victims and their mothers, who saw no reason to break up the family in this way. In Hamilton's case, however, there were compelling motives for getting him out of the house. There were a large number of these prep schools distributed along the South Coast at that time. The small town of Seaford, alone, had over a hundred of them. Some were very good, but many had been set up by a business-minded headmaster with no particular educational qualifications, more of a proprietor than an educator, often supported by a hard-working wife who acted as combined matron, secretary and teacher of the junior classes, and by a collection of assistant masters and mistresses, some of them dedicated teachers but usually including various sorts of social misfits and, as is clear from later accounts of the inmates, a fair quota of paedophiles. The recruitment process was totally controlled by the small London firm of Messrs Gabbitas and Thring, a partnership whose smooth working was somewhat impaired through the long-standing mutual detestation that existed between its two members.

Although there were many prep schools in Brighton, it was decided to send young Hamilton back to Southport to board, presumably because of Dr Bailey's previous connections. with the town. The school chosen was "Durley" (Principal Mr D. Herridge), and Hamilton seems to have been happy there, according to the fragmentary recollections of a fellow pupil. It seems that Mr Herridge was a likeable and conscientious man, but we have no accurate record of the school's standard nor of its staffing, and it has long since disappeared.

Ramsgate

Suitably prepared by Durley, Hamilton was sent on to St Lawrence College, Ramsgate (Figure 1.3), where he arrived in 1904. We have ample records of this school, which still flourishes. St Lawrence's was a religious foundation that had started in 1879, some twenty years before Bailey arrived. An address given by the first headmaster, the Reverend E. C. d'Auquier, recorded the early years of the school and gives a flavour of the institution.

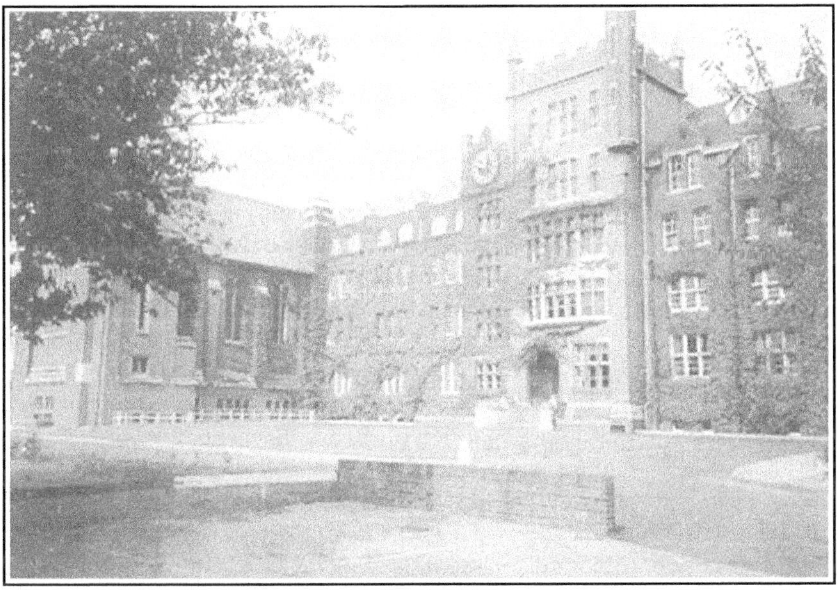

Figure 1.3: St Lawrence College, Ramsgate

> *The instruction given in the school continues on a satisfactory footing. Every pupil is expected to read his Bible morning and evening, and to kneel by his bedside for a few moments before beginning the day's work or retiring to rest. In addition to this, we have the ordinary morning family prayers, at which all the masters and servants are present. The first half-hour of every day is devoted to the study of the Bible. The boys learn a few verses by heart, repeat them, and a short explanation or exhortation arising from the text is then given.*
>
> *The Greek Testament class for the older boys, held by myself, meets three times a week. A new feature this term, which I feel sure will be appreciated, is the intro*

duction of Hebrew.

Perhaps a word about our Staff of Masters may not be uninteresting. Including myself, we now have five Masters of Arts of Cambridge or Oxford, two London Graduates, two English masters, who are about to proceed to their degree, two French and German masters, one of whom is a BA-es Ll., and two music and drawing masters.

In addition to the secular education, great attention continues to be given to physical training. Cricket, football, tennis, tricycling, swimming, have been in full activity; and a look at our boys will convince anyone that the healthiness of the body is considered no less than that of the mind. (Cheers)

We have also lately introduced a Debating Society, which gives promise of good speakers in the future. The library has been enriched by the addition of many volumes for Sunday and week-day reading.

A high moral and spiritual standard is observable among the boys, and the senior boys' influence in the school is all that I could desire. (Cheers)

St Lawrence's was typical of the semi-private institutions that were springing up all round England at that time. These represented a middle ground of education, created by the demands of the upwardly mobile semi-professional classes, who while dissatisfied with the facilities offered by the Board and parochial schools were at the same time unable to afford the fees demanded by the more prestigious places such as Eton, Winchester, Rugby and Marlborough. As with the prep schools, the South Coast, which was recognised to be bracing and healthy, abounded in this type of school, which offered boarding facilities for pupils from the cities and more "relaxing" parts of the country, but at the same time depended heavily on the local population to provide them with day pupils.

Hamilton Bailey was a pupil at St Lawrence's from Michaelmas Term 1908 to Summer Term 1910. He was in the Dark Red House of which the Housemaster was Mr W. Longbourne-Smith ("Dark Red" referred not to the brickwork but rather to the colour coding of the group of pupils under Mr Longbourne Smith's benevolent guidance. They all wore dark red caps and blazers). His intellectual development is not recorded, but he does not seem to have distinguished himself academically. In fact, when Dr Bailey told the headmaster that Hamilton wished to become a doctor, the response was that the boy did not have the brains for it. It also seems unlikely that he was much affected by the efforts of the school to direct him into the correct spiritual pathways, as in later life he seldom went to church and while not taking up a stance with free-thinkers and atheists, he seemed quite devoid of any religious beliefs. Rather surprisingly, however, he retained in later life the capacity to quote long passages from the Bible, giving accurate chapter and verse numbers, and only St Lawrence, with its strong exegetic tradition, could have given him this fund of knowledge.

Hamilton was large for his age and an excellent swimmer. The school record of 1905 recorded him as first in the one length competition and in July 1910 he won the three lengths race in the school swimming sports and was junior deep sea swimming champion of the South Coast. This is an impressive title, but there is no record of the rules of the competition or how many entered it in that year. He certainly did not swim the Channel. Around this time, he developed a keen interest in photography, which was rather unusual in the early years of the century, and found a fellow enthusiast in the school, with whom he exchanged cameras. This hobby was very useful to him in later life.

In many respects, it seems that Bailey led a fairly undistinguished career at St Lawrence, and at times was argumentative and difficult. At the end of one term he had accumulated so much detention that one of the masters had to remain at the school for the first few days of the holidays to supervise his work. Given the circumstances of his father's practice in Brighton, it is quite possible that Hamilton did not feel this prolongation of the term as much of a penance. Margaret Bailey was a tempestuous and unpredictable wife and mother, and 100 Rugby Road, with the unspoken presence of his mentally injured sister, and James Bailey's preoccupation with his busy practice, was no a haven of peace for an adolescent. Holidays were quite often spent with Aunt Edith, Margaret's sister, a calm and secure person with no children of her own, who was very fond of him. His departure from the school is recorded in the St Lawrence valete notes for 1910, with no qualifying comment.

Chapter 2
MEDICAL STUDENT

The London Hospital

Early on during his time at St Lawrence, undeterred by the Headmaster's disparaging comments, Hamilton had decided that he would follow his father into the medical profession. Dr Bailey sent him to a private coach to prepare for the College of Preceptors examination at the University of Durham, equivalent to the 1st MB, which would give him the right to be known as "a perpetual student". He passed this at the second attempt, which enabled him to enter the London Hospital Medical College on May 1 1912, being awarded the first MB certificate from Durham a year later in June 1913. The Durham authorities have no record of his name, so that he was probably living at home in Brighton at the time, and working as an external student.

The entrance fee to the Medical College was £21, and an additional arrival fee, of £31.10s, was paid on 14 May. Presumably these amounts were met by Dr Bailey, but Hamilton's living expenses were not generously supported, as he was allowed only £2 a week to cover all expenses in London. We are not sure of where he lodged, but one of his student notebooks has an address in Hampstead on the flyleaf, so perhaps he at one time lived there. Even by the standards of the time, £2 a week was not a sum that enabled a young man to afford much luxury.

The London Hospital, now the Royal London, founded in 1745, was much the largest hospital in the capital, and served, and still serves, a crowded and deprived area in the East End (Figure 2.1). Although there were other hospitals in the neighbourhood (Mile End, St Andrew's Bow, St Mary's Plaistow, St George's in the East), it was to The London that the East Enders gave their particular loyalty and faith, and it provided them with a magnificent service. As in New York, the local population had been enriched by waves of immigrants, in this case the French Huguenots in the 18th century, Eastern European Jews in the 19th, and Pakistanis and Bangladeshis today. The London Hospital has always been a generous receiver of sick people, regardless of race or provenance.

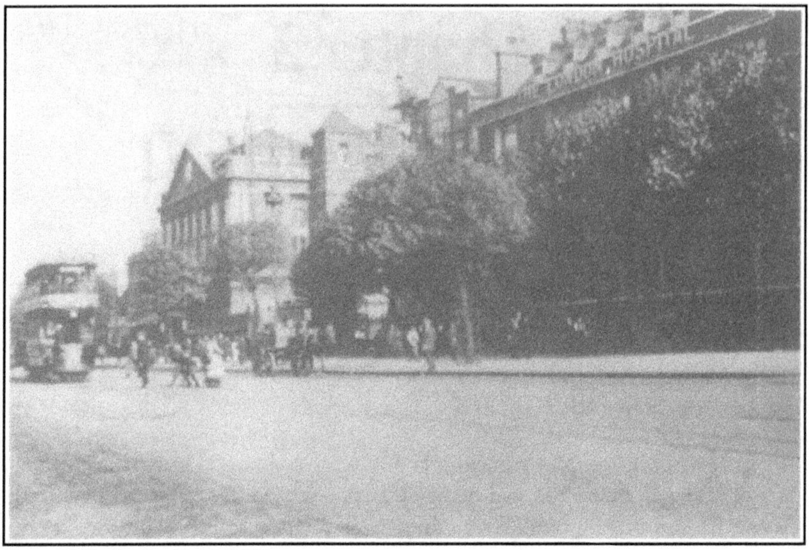

Figure 2.1: The London Hospital, 1904

At the same time, there was a huge social divide between the patients and those who looked after them. The London Hospital nurses, following the Florence Nightingale tradition, tended to be well-established young ladies. The most famous of them, Edith Cavell, who composed the wonderful phrase "Patriotism is not enough..." as she faced the German firing squad on a cold Brussels dawn in 1915, was the refined daughter of a Norfolk manor house. The students and young doctors from whom the future consultants were recruited, for the most part came from professional and middle-class families, and some of them were very rich. They modelled themselves on the consultant staff, who were seen as clear examples of success, power and affluence. There was a well-defined pecking order. The ideal to be aimed at was a post as a general physician or surgeon, at one's own or, even better, at someone else's teaching hospital (a goal scored away from home is always worth more). Next in the hierarchy of eminence were the specialists in orthopaedics, gynaecology, dermatology and so forth, but to end up as a mere general practitioner was, as Lord Moran was later to express it, "to have slipped off the ladder", a verbal slip on his part which many years later helped to destroy his reputation and to rekindle interest in primary care. Appointment as an Honorary (unpaid) consultant at one of the major London Teaching Hospitals was a tremendous privilege, hotly competed for, and a hospital of the calibre and distinction of The London could be sure to attract a talented surgical staff. Not only was such a post a mark of prestige, but it also afforded a wide experience in treating a mass of uncomplaining and docile patients who, as the Honorary was giving his services free, were expected to be duly appreciative. Ironically, the poorer and more populous the charitable district, the greater was the range of instructive cases and hence its usefulness to the private practitioner, a fact not lost on the more observant and ambitious students. It followed that those doctors who had arrived at the top had every incentive to draw up the ladder, and to be wary of any arrival with new and potentially dangerous ideas.

At the time that Hamilton joined as a student, the three outstanding surgeons at The London were Sir Hugh Lett, Sir Henry Souttar and Sir Frederick Treves. These were all remarkable, and remarkably different, characters. Hugh Lett was a slim delicately featured surgical artist, famous for his intricate work on the thyroid gland. Henry Souttar was a mechanical genius, constantly inventing new techniques and instruments, and ever looking for new fields to conquer with his innovative techniques. He was the first to devise a flexible tube to be introduced through a cancer of the throat, which enabled the victims to swallow. Constant coughing and spluttering of food and liquids, and even of one's own saliva, is a miserable indignity, and Souttar's tube (which is still in use today) was a blessing to people with this common and very unpleasant disease. It is not so well known that he was also the first surgeon to operate electively on the heart. One day, passing through the post mortem room, he saw the exposed chest of a young man who had died from a narrowed mitral valve. "Why is that heart so big?" he asked, and was told that the outlet had closed down so that the blood could not escape, and the pump had dilated and failed. "But that is a surgical problem, there is obstruction", replied Souttar, and subsequently persuaded the physicians to allow him to operate on another man with the same type of heart condition, dilating the valve with his finger, and producing a spectacular relief. The man survived for many years, but so envious were his non-surgical colleagues that he was never allowed to operate on another case.

But of the three, undoubtedly the most powerful and charismatic, and the one who particularly influenced the young Hamilton Bailey, was Sir Frederick Treves (Figure 2.2). Treves had been born at Dorchester in 1853, the son of an upholsterer. He was educated at the Merchant Taylors School and University College London, and entered the London Hospital in 1871, qualifying as LSA in 1874, MRCS in 1875 and FRCS in 1878. He was elected as assistant surgeon to The London in 1879, and full surgeon in 1884. He soon attained fame as a writer and teacher, and as consultant to the Army in South Africa during the Boer War was present at the relief of Ladysmith. Honours followed (CB KCVO in 1901) and in 1902 he was made a hereditary Baronet.

Treves had achieved his reputation and baronetcy by his courageous treatment of the Prince of Wales. Following the death of Queen Victoria in 1901, her son Edward VII was due to be crowned in Westminster Abbey, and all the sovereign heads of Europe had been invited to the ceremony. A few days before the coronation, when everything was in readiness, the new king, who was exceedingly fat, began to feel a severe pain in his right lower abdomen. Various specialists were called in, and eventually it was decided that a surgical opinion should be sought, and Treves was summoned to Buckingham Palace, where he diagnosed a new and hitherto unknown condition called "acute appendicitis" and recommended immediate intervention. It was pointed out to him that this was a most awkward moment to choose to operate on an uncrowned monarch, and that it would be better all round to continue with enemas and poultices. Treves stood his ground and said that unless his advice was followed he could not be responsible for his sovereign's life. The scared physicians retreated and a wooden operating table was brought into the basement of the Palace. With great difficulty Treves drained a life-threatening septic appendix from the depths of the royal abdomen. This was the kind of operation that was to become all too familiar to Bailey in later years. Nowadays such a procedure would be quite simple, even for a surgeon in training, but the difficulties in 1902, given the absence of fluid replacement and antibiotics, and even more importantly of relaxant anaesthetic drugs, which could soften the abdominal wall and simplify the approach, were unimaginable. The price of failure would have been enormous, but the king's life was saved, and reward duly followed. Treves achieved an overnight reputation for courage and diagnostic brilliance, and as well as his baronetcy was appointed Sergeant Surgeon to the King, a post which he held till 1910.

Treves' character comes into brighter focus because of his rescue of Joseph Merrick, the Elephant Man. The story has been made into a play and a film, but is worth telling again as it illustrates other aspects of this remarkable surgeon, who was a major influence on Bailey's early life, although the events took place many years before his arrival at The London.

In 1884, one of the squalid stalls in the Whitechapel Road, opposite the front door of the hospital, exhibited a painting of a deformed creature described as "The Elephant Man", who could be viewed for two pence. Treves' curiosity was aroused and he entered the shop. This is what he described.

> *The showman pulled back the curtain revealing a bent figure couched on a stool, covered with a blanket, and huddled over a Bunsen burner trying to keep warm. "Stand up" called out the showman, and the thing arose slowly, letting the blanket fall. It was naked to the waist. A little man, below average height, the most curious thing about him was his enormous and misshapen head, the circumference of which was equal to that of his waist. From his forehead protruded a huge mass of bone. From the back of it, great folds of spongy skin hung down, looking like a cauliflower. An osseous growth occluded one eye. Another mass of bone protruded from his mouth, everting his upper lip, and it was this which had been exaggerated into an imaginary trunk. His face was as incapable of expression as a mass of knarled wood. Never had I met such a degraded and perverted version of a human being as this lame figure displayed.*

Treves rage and sympathy were aroused. Alone among the gawping crowd, he perceived not a freak exhibit but a suffering fellow human being. He spoke gently to the Elephant Man, gave him his visiting card and paid for a hansom cab to bring him over to the hospital, where he carried out a careful interview and

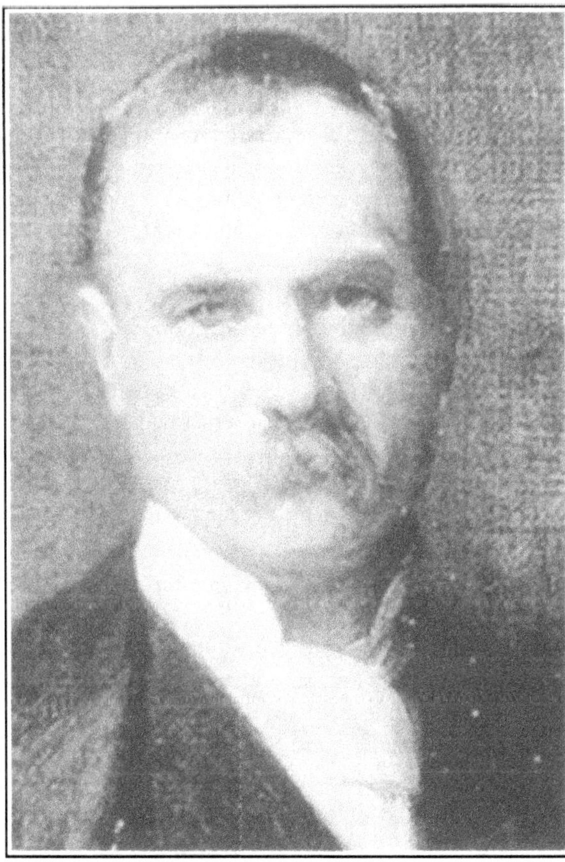

Figure 2.2: Sir Frederick Treves, portrait by Luke Fildes R.A.

physical examination. Treves went back across the Whitechapel Road the next day to find that the exhibition had been closed down by the police and the shopkeeper had decamped with his victim to Brussels in an attempt to evade British law and to exploit the unsupervised Continental market. However, he met with no success in Belgium and a few weeks later sent the wretched Merrick back to London, who arrived at the barrier at Liverpool Street Station with no papers other than an expired rail ticket and Treves' card. Treves was sent for and took the Elephant Man back to the hospital where he found him a small room. Over the next few weeks he worked hard to understand his extraordinary patient and to secure for him the affection and respect he had lacked for the whole of his life. His efforts were rewarded because Merrick was in fact a person of great intelligence, whose speech difficulties were purely the result of deformity and social deprivation, and he soon blossomed. He was taken up by society, invited to the opera and visited by fashionable ladies, including the Princess of Wales, with whom he struck up a friendship. There were even rumours of romantic attachments in high places. Eventually, Merrick died in his sleep from a fractured spine, caused by the enormous weight of his unsupported head. The fact that he perished as a peaceful and happy man was entirely the result of Treves' compassion and understanding.

In 1908, at the age of 52, Treves retired from his hospital appointments to cultivate his vineyard in France, occasionally returning to London to teach the students, carry out an operation when asked to do so and maintain his duties at the Palace, as surgeon to Queen Alexandra and later to George V. He continued in this way until the outbreak of war in 1914.

Bailey was an assiduous student at The London, as his first-year lecture notes on biology and physiology confirm. In spite of his rather mediocre academic performance at St Lawrence, it is clear that he had an exceptional scientific brain, an avidity for information, and a capacity to analyse and record it. He also drew quite well, and his draughtsmanship gives some hint of future surgical dexterity. He was awarded an honorary certificate in minor surgery in 1913, and won the Douro Hoare Physiology Prize in the following year, to the value of £5. This insignificant sum would have been very important because it allowed him to buy necessary bones and textbooks. His clinical reports as an outpatient dresser, and an in-patient dresser under Hugh Lett and Henry Souttar, were reported as "very good", and a note is made that he might make an excellent House Surgeon. All seemed set for a smooth ascent of the medical ladder, throwing away the constraints of his childhood, but larger events were to intervene. Although Bailey worked for Lett and Souttar, and was never Treves' assistant, there can be no doubt that the influence of this towering figure coloured the

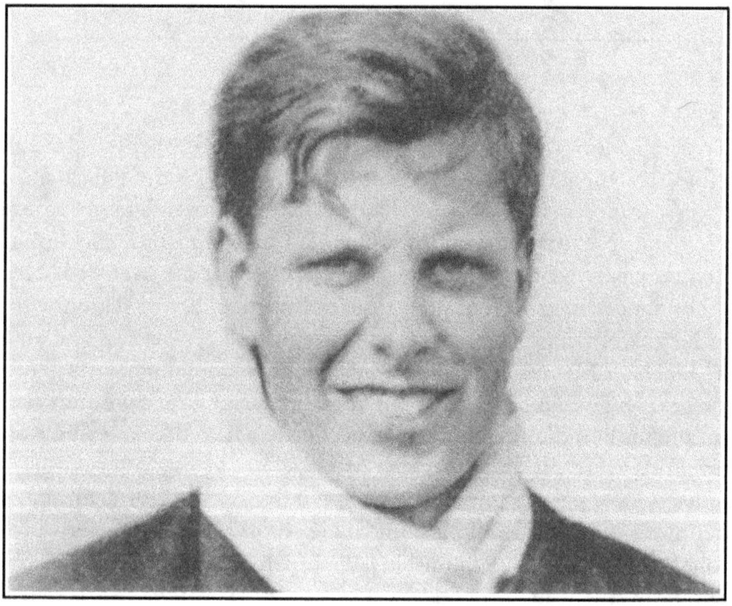

Figure 2.3: Hamilton Bailey as a medical student, 1914

surgical life of the London Hospital at that time, and it was to Treves that Bailey turned in 1914, when the question of his war service became acute.

The First World War

War had broken out between the Allies and the Central European powers earlier in the year, and there was immediate pressure on able bodied young men to join the fighting forces. Bailey was six foot in height, robust, good-looking and athletically built (Figure 2.3).

Although conscription had not been introduced, and medical students were classified as being in a reserved occupation, exempt from enlistment, one can well imagine the comments that were passed in public places on why this conspicuously healthy young man was not volunteering for the Front. Whether because of this sort of pressure, or the influence of his father, or simply natural conscience, in May 1914 he approached Treves and asked to be appointed as a dresser attached to the British Red Cross Mission in Belgium.

Predictably, Treves had involved himself wholeheartedly in the medical support of the Allied Armies. Too old to be given his own command, he joined the Executive Committee of the British Red Cross, and set about organising voluntary help. It was Treves' idea to compose Units that were sent abroad for some special purpose, for example, to staff a hospital or to serve in an ambulance train. A Unit consisted of medical officers, nurses, orderlies, clerks, cooks and dressers. Dressers were responsible for applying pads and bandages to wounds, and were recruited from medical students in their third or fourth year. About 100 of them were sent abroad in the early days of the war, following the previous successful experience that the Red Cross had had with the deployment of students in the Balkan Wars. Later on, the Executive Committee were requested to discontinue the practise of recruiting dressers, and to withdraw those who were already abroad, partly to enable them to continue their hospital studies, and so prevent a future shortage of doctors, but also because, as the war continued, they seemed to be growing less useful, and their somewhat indefinite duties were being carried out more effectively by the trained nurses who were now taking their place in every military hospital. However, in 1914 dressers were still in great demand (it should be remembered that in that year Hamilton Bailey was in his second rather than his third or fourth year of training, so that he must have exerted a degree of deception in getting himself recruited).

Belgium

The First Belgian Unit left Charing Cross Station early on the morning of 15 August 1914, and Bailey was among them. The crossing was rough, but the party was well received at Ostend, and thence went on to Brussels, where they were greeted by a large enthusiastic crowd around the North Station. The Unit was accommodated in the Hotel Astoria, while the local Red Cross Chief, Sir Alfred Keogh, looked around for a suitable site for a base hospital in the neighbourhood of Malines. For the time being, there semed very little for the Unit to do.

Three days after their arrival, a Belgian Count turned up at the hotel in a car flying the Red Cross, and requested the names of two surgeons who would volunteer to go to an outlying village which was under bombardment. Captains Austin and Elliott collected a few instruments and set off. They never came back. A few days later, the driver returned and explained that Austin and Elliott had been captured by the Germans and their car commandeered. The Chief of the Red Cross Unit, Dr Wyatt of St Thomas', got in touch with the American Embassy to try and secure their release, but was told that nothing could be done. It later transpired that the pair were still alive, having been interned in Königsberg Fortress near Hamburg.

Back in London, Treves was furious. He explained to the Executive Committee of the BRCS that the capture of these Red Cross personnel was in direct contravention of Article 9 of the Geneva Convention, and described many other actions of the German Army representing similar breaches. He went on to report frustration on the part of the Society's Unit in Belgium, who had had no wounded soldiers to care for, and had been reduced to moving food supplies. Instead of being a help to the Belgians, Treves felt that they might even run the risk of becoming a burden. The Unit was now joined by eight nurses from the St John's Ambulance Association, who were unsupported in Brussels, their Commission having left. In spite of every effort on the part of the Society to provide the combined group with funds, money began to run out. Things now went from bad to worse. A few weeks after the arrival of the Unit there were rumours that Liège had fallen, and that the central column of the German Army was drawing near. The inhabitants of Brussels were greatly alarmed, and although the authorities assured them of the imminent arrival of a relieving French Force, there was no certainty of this. Nobody seemed to be in overall control, and people began to desert the capital.

One morning, Bailey and his Unit woke up to find that all the Belgian soldiers in Brussels had left for Antwerp, and a few hours later the German troops began to march into the city. Over the next three days, a continuous stream of men and vehicles poured through. The windows of the Hotel Astoria were blockaded with mattresses; and food supplies became scarce. The German garrison quickly established some sort of order, and as soon as the Red Cross Unit was identified they were turned out of their comfortable billet in the Astoria, which was given over to the occupying troops, and sent to Schaerbeek Station (Schaerbeek is a suburb in northern Brussels; Figure 2.4) to attend to the wounded captives on their way to Germany. Rooms at the station were turned into a casualty clearing station, and as the trains passed through, the medical teams, who did alternate day and night dutys, fed and dressed the prisoners. Only the most seriously wounded

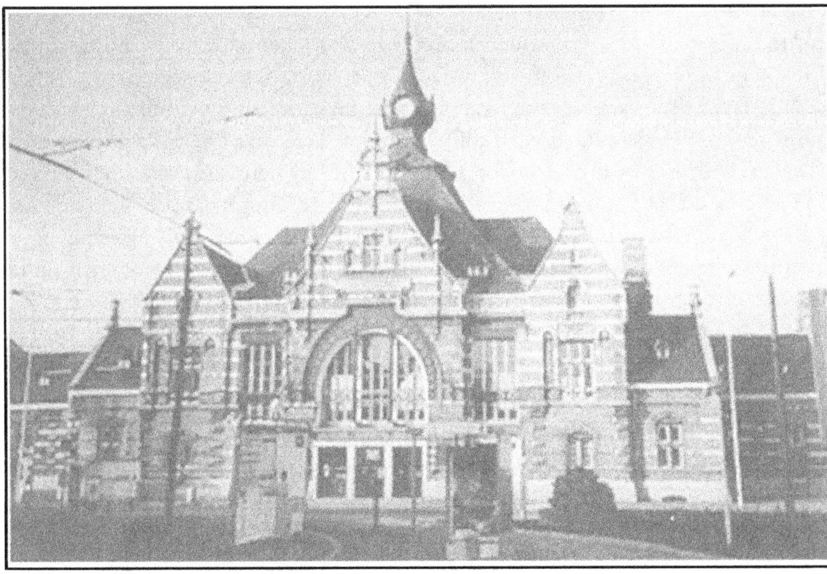

Figure 2.4: Schaerebeek Station, outside Brussels

were allowed to leave the trains. Some of the victims of the Mons campaign were in a dreadful state, their wounds not having been dressed since a Field Bandage had been hurriedly applied as much as a week previously. One day a large number of civilians from Louvain arrived to be fed, two of whom appeared to have become completely demented. Bailey and his friends tied up their hands and feet and obtained permission to send them to a mental asylum in Brussels. However, one slight concession was gained in that one of the Society's surgeons and two of the nurses were allowed to attend the railway station night and day, to obtain the home addresses of British Prisoners of War as they passed through, each medical officer having his own list. As a result, the Red Cross was able to send many letters to the families of missing soldiers in Britain, confirming that they were still alive.

This existence continued for about seven weeks, until November 1914. Bailey wrote to his parents in Brighton that "the English prisoners accepted their fate sulkily, while the Frenchmen gave themselves over entirely to grief. We had no news except the German Proclamations, which could always be summed up as unmitigated success all along their line". At the end of this period, the party was split up, some of the nurses being sent to the ruined town of Charleroi. The money was almost gone, but a kindly solicitor lent them a house near to the station, and they were able to subsist on small advances from the Belgian Red Cross. Luckily, there was also living in the house a young American woman who was working for the United States Embassy and who befriended the group.

One day Hamilton found that his boots were disintegrating, and he walked into the centre of Brussels to have them repaired. On the way back, he was arrested by a private detective, who was unsatisfied by the state of his papers, and turned him over to the German forces. He was taken at bayonet point to the local depot, and placed before a summary Court Martial as a suspected spy. "When at length the time came for me to appear", he says, "it was my misfortune to have to go along a passage lined with soldiers. It was here that I became unpleasantly familiar with the butt end of the German rifle". Then came the questioning, "How was it that I was in possession of Sir Edward Grey's passport?" (The mistake was understandable. Grey was the Foreign Secretary, and in those days, every British passport carried the Minister's name.) "Why did I not own up to the fact that I had come over in a troopship?" Vainly protesting, he was marched off to the local German War Headquarters. On the way, two other members of the Unit, Croft and Robinson, who happened to be in the street, recognised Bailey and hailed him enthusiastically, which resulted in their being immediately put under arrest and joining the march. The interview with a German officer was polite, but they were nonetheless imprisoned on suspicion. They shared a cell with a group of suspected spies including two young men, a Belgian and Frenchman. A few days after their arrival these two were called out by the guards and Bailey and his friends watching through the window saw them driven away by a party of soldiers. The car returned containing the escort, but with no passengers. The German guards explained that they had been found guilty of espionage and had been shot on the outskirts of the town, and that the turn of the remaining prisoners, including Bailey, was coming soon. The effect of this message on the morale of the cell's occupants is easy to imagine.

However, the young American woman had not forgotten her group of friends. Prompted by her, the United States Ambassador intervened, demanding that all British medical students and nurses should be repatriated, under the terms of the Geneva Convention. The Unit was temporarily freed, and left Brussels, but got only as far as Liège, where they were re-arrested and sent back to jail. Once more the American Minister providentially intervened, this time with success. The Unit was sent from Liège to Aix-la-Chapelle, and then on to Cologne. On arrival in Germany, they were jeered at and set upon by the populace, and only the intervention of the local American Consul saved them from serious assault. The following four days were passed in a fourth-class carriage travelling through Germany to Denmark. The train travelled at five or ten miles an hour and sleep was impossible owing to the number of people in the carriage, none of whom was able to lie down.

Bailey recounts the one break in the journey, in Schleswig-Holstein, when they were allowed out of the train to wash at a village pump. It was a most delicious refreshment, in spite of the fact that rifles were pointed at him from every direction. His typically understated comment was that "it was a most trying journey".

At last, the frontier was crossed, and an immediate sense of joy and liberation was experienced by the captives. Suddenly the atmosphere changed and the bleak Holstein countryside was replaced by the red roofed cottages, storks, hollyhocks and geraniums of southern Denmark. As the train rattled on across the islands and ferries into Copenhagen station, spirits rose, and there was a great welcome awaiting them. The British Embassy was aware of the arrival of the party, and made every effort to make up for their previous privations. During their week in Copenhagen, they were fêted by both the Danes and the English community. Bailey visited the National Hospital (Rigshospitalet) and was impressed with its elaboration and modernity. They dined in the Residents' quarters, and met two young doctors, Petersen and Hennes, who had studied at the London. Another most important contact was with Dr Carl Krebs, at that time a young Resident at the Rigshospitalet, who immediately developed a fellow feeling with Bailey, which was reciprocated, and during his brief stay took pains to show him as much as he could of Danish medicine. This was the start of a friendship that was to last for 50 years. Krebs was later to become an eminent figure in the Danish medical world, as the first Professor of Radiology, and Director of Services in Aarhus. Following a week in Denmark, the party travelled via Sweden to Bergen, where they were joined by the crew of an English merchant ship which had been torpedoed by a German submarine. Eventually, after a rough crossing of the North Sea, they steamed into Newcastle on the 23 October 1914. "We were in the Mother country once more."

Hamilton Bailey's story, which appeared in the *London Hospital Gazette* for December 1914, is a composed and mature, almost phlegmatic, account of the what one would have thought to have been a terrifying few weeks for a young student. He seems never to have feared for his own life, which had obviously been at great risk. Part of this could be ascribed to the arrogant self-confidence of young middle-class Englishmen of the time, accustomed as they were to despise foreigners, rule large numbers of subject people, and have total trust in the universal efficacy of the British passport. Did he realise that he might quite easily have been executed by the Germans, or died of typhus or of starvation in some remote North European railway siding ? If so, it does not come across in this account. One is tempted to speculate that a lack of affection in his family life had inured him to negative experiences. He did not expect to be loved or even liked or appreciated. He might, perhaps, have felt the need to be respected. In all this record there is no hint or suggestion of self pity or indeed of self regard. At the same time, however, although the sense of duty and obligation towards the sick and wounded is very clear, concern and compassion, although perhaps felt, are not much in evidence.

Back in London

In 1915, Britain, with a population of 45 million, had 700,000 men at the Front, whilst France, where conscription had been introduced at the beginning of the War, with 40 million inhabitants, had 2.5 million men on active service. Although at first voluntary recruitment had worked well, as the year went by, figures for enlistment actually fell, and there was a growing demand for compulsory military service to be brought in. This was, however, opposed in the Cabinet, most particularly by Lord Kitchener, the hero of Omdurman, who was by now Secretary of State for War, and who had always believed in the principle of a voluntary army, and in the feasibility of raising the millions of troops necessary to defeat the Germans, through voluntary means. Nobody else thought it remotely possible. Under pressure from the French, and as the need for men became more urgent, Kitchener's supporters in Cabinet gradually gave way. A National Register was established in July 1915, and in October a Manchester business man, Lord Derby, was put in charge of a new scheme for stimulating recruitment. The Derby Scheme provided that all men between the ages of 18 and 21 should be asked to "attest", i.e. to volunteer for active service as soon as their year was called up. These men were known as Derby Recruits, and it was a group of them who spotted Bailey, recently returned from captivity by the Germans, sitting peacefully on top of an open double-decker bus under the railway bridge at Bethnal Green in East London. Seeing him dressed in civilian clothes and struck by his health and stature, they shouted insults at him, crying out, "why aren't you in khaki, you slacker ?". A young woman dashed up the stairs of the bus and delighted the passengers by producing from her handbag a white feather, the accepted mark of cowardice, which she presented to Bailey with an exaggerated curtsey. (There was a certain type of woman around London at that time who never left home without a supply of white feathers, in case of such opportunities.) There were shouts of applause. Bailey's reaction is not recorded.

Incidentally, the Derby Scheme soon proved a complete failure, and when compulsory military service was introduced the following year Lord Derby resigned in disgust and could only be consoled by being put in charge of the Air Force, a post which his colleagues induced him to relinquish after a few months.

The medical student record of the London Hospital Medical College goes on to record that Bailey passed the second Conjoint Board in January 1915 and the first Conjoint Board in Pharmacy the following October. He failed the Primary FRCS examination at the first attempt. Apart from the Durham MB, this was the only examination he ever failed, and his mother's comments are unrecorded. (He subsequently passed the Primary in September 1919.) He was awarded the James Anderson Prize in Elementary Clinical Medicine (with a value of £2) in 1915, and went on to be dresser to Mr Frank Kidd in the Genitourinary Surgical Outpatients during the latter part of that year. This was followed by a period of dresser to the Special Department, which in fact was the department of venereal, or as we would now say sexually transmitted diseases. Such was the sense of guilt and shame associated with these infections that the place where they were treated never alluded to directly, but simply referred to as "The Special Department". His clinical clerkship under Dr Robert Hutches (a medical as opposed to a surgical apprenticeship) was recorded as "good". In August 1916 he obtained the Licentiate of Medicine and Surgery of the Society of Apothecaries, which made him a doctor.

The Navy

From here on one would expect a quiet transfer from adventure in Germany to resumed medical studies in wartime London, but in fact things did not work out like this. In 1915 Hamilton volunteered for service in the Royal Navy. Knowing his character, it is unlikely that the incident on the Bethnal Green bus in any way influenced his decision. The reactions of James and Margaret are not recorded, but one would suspect that James at least approved, from what we know of him. He had, after all, served at the Naval Hospital in Devonport, before going to Nablus. Now a final-year student, Hamilton was posted to join the Grand Fleet at Scapa Flow in Orkney, with the rank of Temporary Sub-Lieutenant RNVR.

The war situation in 1916, when Bailey had returned to the London, was unfavourable to the Germans. They had lost many troops at Verdun, there were economic problems at home and the recent mid-Atlantic sinking of the *Lusitania*, which was full of women and children, had been received very badly in America, where the Government was on the point of joining the Allied cause. It was politically and militarily urgent for Germany to achieve a convincing victory, and the most obvious front was that of the sea. The theatre in which this drama was to be played out was the west coast of Denmark — Jutland, the land of the Jutes which Bailey had left so triumphantly the year before. The battle of Jutland was not only one of the turning points of the 1914–1918 war, but also a pivotal event in British history, of which the young Bailey was a witness. This was its background.

In October 1805, Horatio Nelson had destroyed the navies of France and Spain at the battle of Trafalgar. For the next century, the Royal Navy was unchallenged and Britain could use sea power to impose her model of trade-based colonisation on the rest of the world. But this stable state of affairs degenerated into rigidity and complacency. The Navy had become preoccupied with spit and polish, precedence and protocol: it was a well-ordered machine designed to rule a peaceful empire. Other nations had quite different views on the Pax Britannica. The German Navy Laws of 1898 and 1900 were designed to create a powerful rival to match Britain's strength. The only man on the British side to appreciate the coming danger was the extraordinary Jackie Fisher, one of the most unlikely people ever to have held the office of First Sea Lord (whose biography has been written by Jan Morris). A little like Nelson, in that he was slight in build, vain, and endlessly energetic, he arrived in the Navy without money, friends or support, and succeeded in climbing that immensely complicated and snobbish organisation by means of unchallengeable competence and a total refusal to accept received ideas. He was described as a mixture of man and child, "remorseless, ruthless and relentless". He revised the naval career structure, finally rid the service of its romantic preoccupation with sail, but above all developed the concept of the battle cruiser, a ship with the fire power of a capital battleship and the manoeuvrability of a cruiser. By the time that war broke out in 1914, Fisher had to an extent succeeded in modernising the Royal Navy's Grand Fleet, although its larger ships were slower, and its guns less powerful and mobile, than their German equivalents. Ironically, German optics were so superior that both sides observed each other through Zeiss lenses manufactured in Jena.

On 30 May 1916 a coded message ("312 Gg 1490") was intercepted by the Admiralty indicating that the German High Seas Fleet was moving out of Wilhelmshaven. At that time, the Grand Fleet was in Scapa Flow, Invergordon and Rosyth. The Commander in Chief was Fisher's protégé, the 57-year-old Sir John Jellicoe, the son of a merchant navy master of marine, small, precise, bespectacled, ascetic, physically disciplined, labelled by many of his juniors as a bureaucrat (his later incursion into Bailey's life at the Royal Northern Hospital is recorded in Chapter 4). Jellicoe's flagship was the *Iron Duke*, to which young Sub-Lieutenant Bailey was assigned as a junior medical officer. The *Iron Duke* weighed 30,000 tons and was one of the most modern battleships in the Navy, carrying ten 13.5-inch guns.

In command of the battle cruiser squadron was a totally contrasting figure, Sir David Beatty, swashbuckling, bold, careless in dress, affable and with a notable combat record. By a strange coincidence, this situation was reflected on the other side. In command of the High Seas Fleet was Grand Admiral Reinhard von Scheer, very much in the Jellicoe mould. Beneath him was Admiral Hipper, a genial and blustering figure not unlike Beatty.

The two armadas slowly closed in, each being in total ignorance of the other's whereabouts. Bearing in mind that radio communication was rudimentary, that visibility in the North Sea was frequently less than a few yards, that messages were still sent between ships by means of flags run up on a masthead, and that many of the sailors were illiterate, it is not surprising that things went badly wrong. A preliminary skirmish between Beatty and Hipper took place to the south of Jutland, at which the battle cruiser *Indefatigable* was sunk. Messages exchanged between Beatty in the Skagerrak and Jellicoe in Orkney, were either not received or misinterpreted, but late on the 30 May 1916 the Grand Fleet sailed southwards. The British were aware that the entire German High Seas Fleet was out of its base, but did not know where it was, whereas the German fleet thought that Beatty's force was the only one in the area and had no idea that the entire might of the Grand Fleet was steaming towards it. Beatty turned north to meet Jellicoe, but because of confused messages, Jellicoe was 7 miles off course and Beatty 4 miles, so that they missed each other by a total of 11 miles. But eventually the fleets met.

When the definitive battle of Jutland was finally joined, the result was confusion and carnage. A Captain Joel had both legs blown off in front of his junior officers; a rating was seen carrying the severed head of one of his comrades. The MO in *Princess Royal* recorded "we treated several cases of burns occurring amongst members of fire repair parties...a gunlayer from the after turret had a foot nearly blown off...later I amputated his leg...I could not bear to imagine what conditions were like below..." In the *Iron Duke*, Bailey was below. The record of his experience on that day is indirect, because he never spoke of it except to his old Danish friend Carl Krebs, to whom he confided that the sick bay was in the "bowels of the ship" and that when the first shot was received all the electric lights went out, the emergency lighting failed and he spent 20 hours in an improvised reception area. Unable to know how the battle was going, and prepared from minute to minute for the ship to receive a direct hit, with no possible chance of escape, he received a succession of mutilated sailors coming down the chute in sacks, and did the best he could for them, which was probably not very much. As a temporary lieutenant he was low down in the chain of command and was there to obey orders rather than to take decisions, but the effect of such an experience on a 20-year-old must have been profound.

When his flagship, the *Lützow*, was destroyed, Hipper was rowed from ship to ship in search of a new place for his Admiral's pennant, at last reaching the *Seydlitz*, which consented to be the centre of command. Following the loss of several cruisers, von Scheer finally realised that the odds were against him and gave orders to withdraw towards Horns Reef, a sandbank which lay across the entrance to the Jade River and Wilmhelmshaven. There was an opportunity for an interception ("crossing the T"), but this was missed by the Allies. For some strange reason, Scheer rescinded his order and turned back to the North, straight into the course of the Grand Fleet. In the engagement which followed the German losses were heavy, but the Royal Navy lost the battle cruisers *Queen Mary*, *Indefatigable*, *Invincible*, *Defence*, *Black Prince* and *Warrior*, together with the destroyers; *Tipperary*, *Turbulent*, *Fortune*, *Sparrowhawk* and *Ardent*, plus sixothers. The *Iron Duke*, with Bailey on board, received many casualties but was not herself in the thick of the action, and escaped damage. At the end of 31 May the fleets disengaged, and limped back to port.

Both sides claimed victory. The Germans declared that "the gigantic fleet of Albion which since Trafalgar has imposed on the whole world a brand of sea tyranny...has been humiliated". The British communiqué was more factual, and limited itself to enumerating the losses. In fact, the crippled German High Seas Fleet never again put to sea, so to that extent Jutland was an Allied success. But the price paid was high, not only in terms of losses of men and material, but also because the myth of British naval supremacy was finally exploded.

The *Iron Duke* with Bailey on board returned to Scapa Flow. At that time he was still a student, but in August 1916 he obtained the Licentiate of the Society of Apothecaries which made him a fully qualified doctor. There was no compulsory internship or pre-registration year at that time, so that without further experience he was automatically promoted into the RN, with the rank of Surgeon Lieutenant (Figure 2.5), carrying a single stripe on his sleeve, bordered in red, to indicate that he was not a proper sailor, but rather one of the Senior Service's necessary supporters. Still in the Navy, Bailey returned to the London Hospital where on 30 October 1916 he was appointed as House Surgeon to Messrs Hugh Rigby and Robert Milne, a job he continued until January 1917. Presumably this was to enable him to gain more clinical experience before resuming his active service at the Royal Naval Hospital at Plymouth. From June 1917 he served in a rather unusual type of ship, the "monitor" *M19*, a hybrid type of vessel used only in the two world wars. Intended for coastal bombardment, it combined a small hull with a very large gun (in the case of *M19*, 540 tons with a 9.2-inch gun). Life in such a confined space must have had its problems, but *M19* was based in the Mediterranean, well outside the theatre of war, so that this period of his service was comparatively relaxed and agreeable, though no personal records have survived. This was his last time at sea. His subsequent naval career was not entirely happy. On being posted back to Scapa Flow, this time as a Medical Officer to the German Navy, he had to deal with a major influenza epidemic. His request for the use of a motor launch to visit the sick was refused by his superiors, whereupon Bailey wired a complaint direct to the Admiralty. Not surprisingly, his Commanding Officer was furious at this flagrant breach of discipline, but, as his period of service was coming to an end, he escaped a Court Martial and was sent back to Portsmouth. Here, there was a last flash of success, described in Bailey's own words.

> *On Armistice night 1918, I was transferred from the Royal Naval Barracks Portsmouth to the Royal Naval Hospital Edinburgh to take the place of a physician who became struck down by the 1918 'flu epidemic. I was only just 23 years of age and was of course a makeshift for a physician in charge of wards. Next day (my first day of duty) a post captain was admitted to the Officers Block diagnosed as 'flu' I found that he had a perforated gastric ulcer and got the operating surgeon (now senior surgeon at Charing Cross Hospital) along on Saturday afternoon to operate. I gave the anaesthetic! My PMO (surgeon Captain Lindsay) was so pleased with me that he had me placed on the 'permanent' staff of Granton Hospital opposite number to Surgeon Lieutenant Commander Briggs, later editor of the* Royal Naval Medical Journal.

(In fact, official naval records confirm that Bailey was appointed to Granton on November 1918, just before the Armistice, and that Briggs was on the Staff. The name of Lindsay is wrong, but there was a Commander Livesay present at the time, and that is probably a simple transcription error.) Bailey was discharged from the Navy shortly afterwards in 1919, perhaps to the relief of his fellow officers, and returned to The London, where he obtained the LRCP MRCS Conjoint qualification, and the following year passed the final examination for FRCS. The *Iron Duke* continued in service until 1946, when it was sold for scrap.

Humphries says, "he did not enjoy his naval service, and was thankful to obtain his release in 1919 after what had been a boring ordeal". This scarcely meets the case. Three years out of the life of a patriotic young man, who was looking ambitiously at a professional future, might have been seen as a frustrating penance, or even an ordeal, but scarcely boring, if one includes caring for the wounded at a historic naval battle, cruising the Mediterranean in a small ship, looking after the sailors of a defeated enemy and as a result narrowly missing disgrace at a Court Martial.

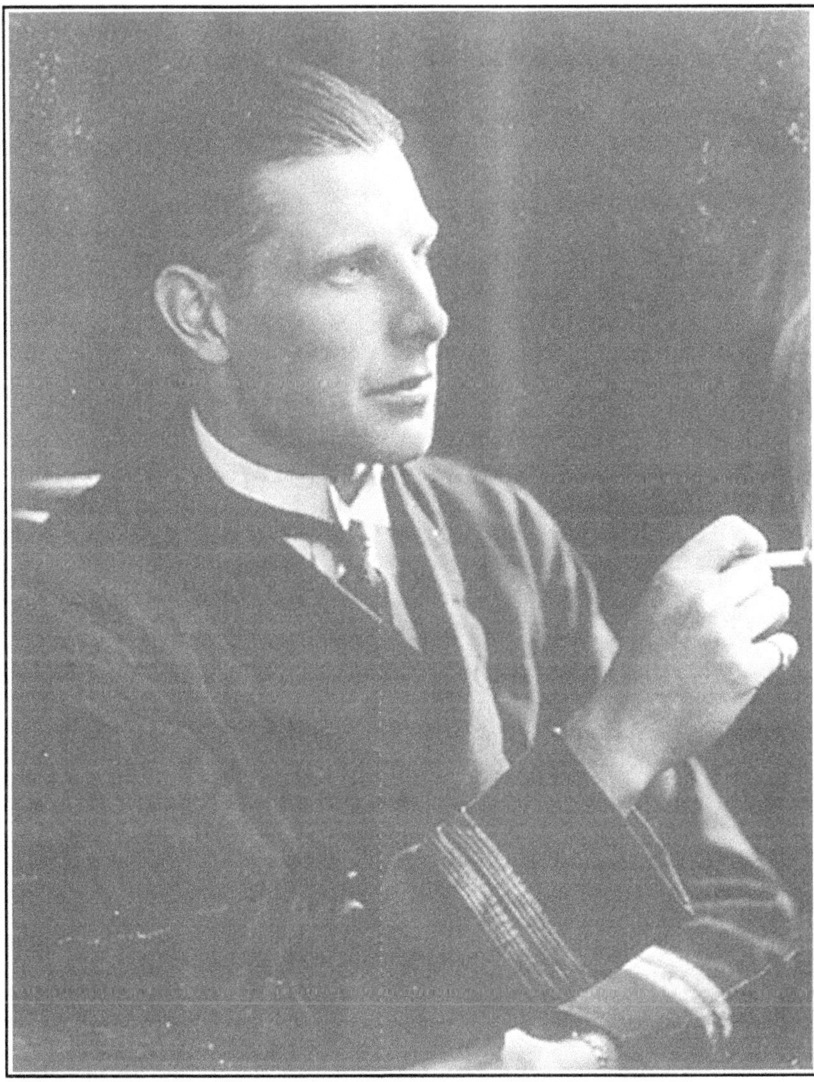

Figure 2.5: Surgeon Lieutenant H. H. Bailey, R N

Chapter 3

THE YOUNG SURGEON

Wolverhampton

Having completed his house appointments, and gained his FRCS, the next logical step was to seek for a post as Registrar to broaden his experience at a higher level of responsibility. There was no immediate prospect of promotion at the London, and Bailey accepted the advice of his seniors to further his training in a provincial hospital with a good reputation and a busy clinical practice. He applied for and was (apparently) appointed to the post of Resident Surgical Officer to Wolverhampton and South Staffordshire General Hospital, which was later to become the Royal Hospital, Wolverhampton. In this appointment, and indeed in other subsequent posts for which Bailey competed, there does seem to have been an element of uncertainty and intrigue. On 7 January 1921 the medical committee interviewed three candidates for the post, and appointed a Mr Pinkerton. Four days later, Pinkerton appeared before the Board of Management for his appointment to be confirmed, but demanded 24 hours notice before agreeing to accept it. This irritated the Board, and their minutes dated 18 January 1921 record that the Chairman, Mr Tom B. Adams, having consulted with the Honorary Surgeons, had appointed Mr Hamilton Bailey FRCS as Resident Surgical Officer in accordance with the terms of the advertisement. The Board duly confirmed the action of the Chairman. Strangely, the minutes of the Medical Committee dated 7 January state 'the Committee had before them the applications for the post of RSO from Messrs Pinkerton, Hamilton Bailey and MacMillan & interviewed the last two. Mr Pinkerton had called on some members of the Staff. The Committee recommended the appointment of Mr Pinkerton'. However the name of Pinkerton is written differently, and it has been suggested that it may have been a later addition. Another version suggests that Mr Pinkerton demanded an even longer period of reflection before accepting the appointment, and that this swayed the Committee in Bailey's favour. Pinkerton has disappeared from history, while Bailey lives on, but whatever the truth of the matter, Bailey's stay at Wolverhampton only lasted for a few months. Shortly after taking up his duties, he had a major disagreement with the Senior Surgeon, Edward Deanesly. The exact point at issue is not known, but Deanesly was a most unwise choice of antagonist. He had spent his entire professional life in Wolverhampton, had been instrumental in building the reputation of the hospital, to which he had donated an excellent pathology department, and was a prominent Town Councillor with a reputation for being opinionated and outspoken. As well as being the major influence in the town's medical affairs, he was an accomplished surgeon with a number of important publications to his credit. From the moment that Bailey aroused Deanesly's disapproval, his future prospects in Wolverhampton vanished.

In June 1921 a Registrar post back at The London fell vacant, and Bailey immediately applied, but to his great disappointment the job was given to a rival, G. E. Neligan. Frustrated at Wolverhampton, he decided to continue his provincial hospital experience further North, and was successful in his application for the post of Surgical Registrar at Liverpool Royal Infirmary. The later Minute Books from Wolverhampton make no mention of Bailey, and it is even possible that he was in a locum post and was never offered the permanent appointment following the row with Deanesly. However, there were no lasting hard feelings, as in the seventh edition of *Emergency Surgery*, which appeared in 1958, Bailey mentions him as 'one of my masters', and includes his photograph. Deanesly's name is still remembered locally, and the recently opened oncology unit is called after him and bears his portrait. His son was a hero of the Second World War. Having joined the RAF in 1937 his Spitfire was twice shot down into the sea but he in turn shot down four German bombers over London in the space of one month in 1941, which earned him a DFC.

Liverpool

Liverpool was a thriving port and industrial city with a large immigrant population, and the Liverpool Royal Infirmary (Figure 3.1), which was closely connected with the Medical School, was one of the most famous teaching centres in Britain, with an especially solid reputation in surgery and orthopaedics, following the pioneering work of Robert Jones, a bluff and determined character who pioneered the treatment of dislocations and fractures through his work in the docks. The staff included Charles Wells (later Professor of Surgery) and Henry Cohen who was to become one of the foremost endocrinologists of the day, and end up as Lord Cohen of Birkenhead, President of the General Medical Council, and still remembered as a brilliant clinician and teacher.

Although skill in the operating theatre is gradually acquired over years of training, most surgeons can recall a defining period which is marked by a sudden surge in self confidence and ability. In later life Bailey always described his Liverpool year as making this transition - a sort of professional puberty. The burden of work was heavy, but the experience gained was invaluable.

Apart from the managing the wards and theatres, the Registrar was expected to take a large share of the undergraduate teaching, and Bailey took up this activity with enthusiasm. Humphries quotes one of his former students as saying:

> *The arrival of Bailey was a godsend and introduced something the like of which we had never seen before. He was a superb teacher of the classical type and we took every advantage of what he could do for us, including coaching classes. We found that in addition to his dedication and enthusiasm for teaching he was extremely sensitive, and even emotional and temperamental. Once, on being told that 'the portal system is formed by the mesenteric and splenic veins (at which stage he looked cheerful and hopeful) joined by the renal vein' he went quite pale, threw his hands up in the air....he ended the class and sent us away, saying that he could not carry on any longer. I have never had any doubts that this was perfectly genuine.*

Dr Ruth Dowy, now in her 95th year, remembers Bailey well and recalls that the female medical students found him an impressive figure and very good looking, as well as being an excellent teacher.

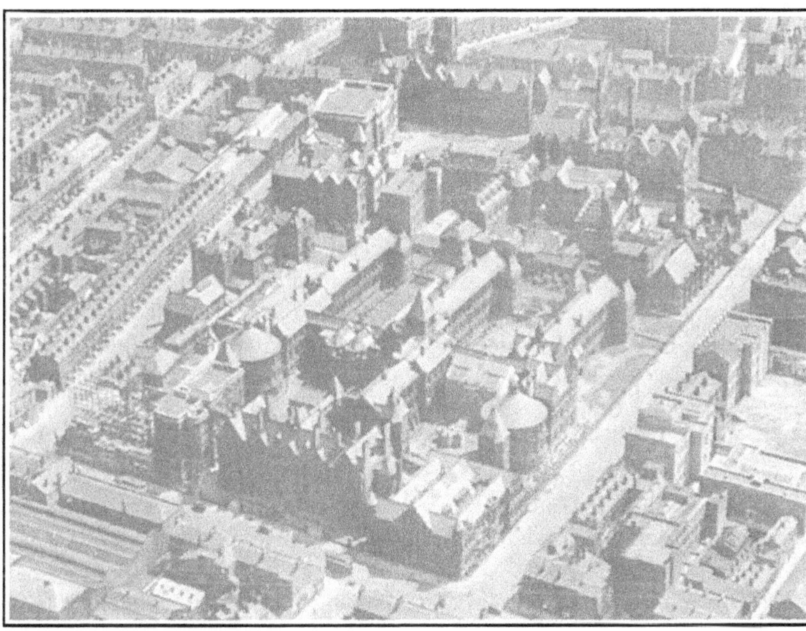

Figure 3.1: The Liverpool Royal Infirmary, 1925

Bailey was not wholly popular in Liverpool, as he was seen as somewhat reserved, supercilious, and pleased with himself. (This is a judgement which the reputedly friendly people of the North of England seem quite often to level against soft spoken competitors from places such as London and Brighton.) In

October 1921 he was enrolled as a country member of the old established and renowned Liverpool Medical Institution, which was certainly a mark of esteem, but there is no record of his attendance. In point of fact Bailey, was, like his father, never at ease socially, disliked cocktail parties and convivial dinners, took no part in any sport and found it difficult to make friends among his contemporaries. He seems to have had little interests outside his work, and spent his free time studying and writing. The first ideas for the series of articles and textbooks were germinating in his mind during this Liverpool year, and there was a positive side to a rather monastic life, in that his careful avoidance of involvement in medical politics meant that while there were not many opportunities for advancement there were at the same time fewer chances of making enemies.

Back to London

At the end of the year, another post at The London became vacant, and Bailey immediately applied. Once again, the appointment was not straightforward. On 23 January 1922 The London Hospital House Committee received the applications for the vacant post of Surgical Registrar. The names of H. H. Bailey, L. G. Brown, G. Hearne, G. Huddy and H. H. Mott were referred to the Medical Council. The leading applicants were Bailey and Brown, and when the Council met on 22 February at the house of Lord Dawson of Penn, at 32 Wimpole Street, they chose Brown, by a majority of 14 to10. However the final authority lay with the House Committee, to whom they had to report. The importance attached to their choice was shown by the seniority of the deputation which they sent to the House Committee, consisting of Lord Dawson, Mr Milne (the senior orthopaedic surgeon) and Mr Openshaw. The House Committee Minute Book records, under Item 9, dated 6 February 1922 that 'the Deputation recommended that Mr L. G. Brown be appointed. However they noted that Mr Brown did not have the qualification of FRCS, which was one of the conditions of the advertisement, and that therefore although they would very much like to have appointed him, they could not agree to the recommendation of the Medical Council. The House Governor was therefore instructed to notify the Secretary of the Council that the Committee appointed Mr Hamilton Bailey to the post, as they understood, officially, that his was the second name recommended by the Medical Council'. This decision was accepted by the Council, as at their meeting a week later the House Committee received a letter from them recommending Bailey, who, they were told, had already been notified of his success.

This episode is recounted in detail, because it is relevant to the story. In the first place, it illustrates the extreme importance attached to the post of Surgical Registrar at a London teaching hospital. Nowadays, there would be fewer applicants, and their candidatures would be considered at a much lower level. It would never occur to a medical member of the House of Lords to call a meeting at his home to discuss such a matter, and then to compose a senior deputation to attend upon a Hospital House Committee, but in the 1920s things were quite different.

Such an appointment was an almost certain guarantee of a successful consultant career, and moreover, as the surgeons did little routine operating in the hospital, and virtually no emergency work, the reputation of the institution depended crucially on the quality of its junior staff. For these reasons, registrar posts were hotly competed for and the applicants were carefully scrutinised. Quite apart from this, the episode tells something of Bailey's personal standing at that time. The Medical Council knew perfectly well that applicants had to possess the FRCS, but instead of choosing the obvious candidate, who was a local product, with the required qualification, an impressive war record and good clinical experience, they instead attempted to persuade the House Committee to break the rules and appoint someone who was clearly ineligible. Bearing in mind his previous unsuccessful application, there must have been some very strong antagonism to Bailey around the London Hospital for its Council to have behaved in this way. We can only speculate on the grounds for this, but the situation was to repeat itself a few years later, with grave results on Bailey's subsequent life.

Bailey was probably quite unaware of what had gone on behind the scenes. He was appointed as Registrar to his old chiefs Hugh Rigby (who had in the meantime earned a Knighthood by operating successfully on the Duke of York, later King George VI) and Robert Milne, who developed the first orthopaedic service at the London. The post was later redesignated as 'First Assistant', but this does not seem to have represented a genuine promotion, but rather an internal rearrangement. The London Hospital First Assistants in 1925 (Figure 3.2) were a brilliant group. They included Russell Brain the neurologist, later President of the Royal College of Physicians, Donald Hunter who created the specialty of occupational medicine, George Huddy, and the neurosurgeon Hugh Cairns, who became the first Nuffield Professor of Surgery at Oxford. Most notable among the group was his friend and competitor Robert McNeill Love, who was later to become a colleague at the Royal Northern Hospital and the co-author of two of his most famous works, the *Short Practice of Surgery* and *Surgery for Nurses*.

The work of a Surgical Registrar at a London hospital in the 1920s was extremely arduous. During their periods of duty, which lasted for up to a week, they worked a 24 hour day, snatching sleep as the opportunity arose. During the daylight hours they assisted the Chief in the operating theatre, wards and clinics, and kept all the medical records. They were expected to attend his ward round and to carry out his instructions to the letter, and to deputise for him when he was away conducting an examination, attending a medical conferences or shooting grouse in Scotland. In addition, they supervised the House Staff and did most of the undergraduate teaching. When the day's work was ended, they continued seeing accident and emergency patients in the Receiving Room, operating on them as required. It was very seldom that a Consultant would be called in to advise (in any case, not all of them were on the telephone) and to summon help would be considered as a mark of immaturity. Not surprisingly, in view of this sort of pressure, things quite often went wrong, but complaints from patients were rare and not well received (after all, it was said, they were getting a free service).

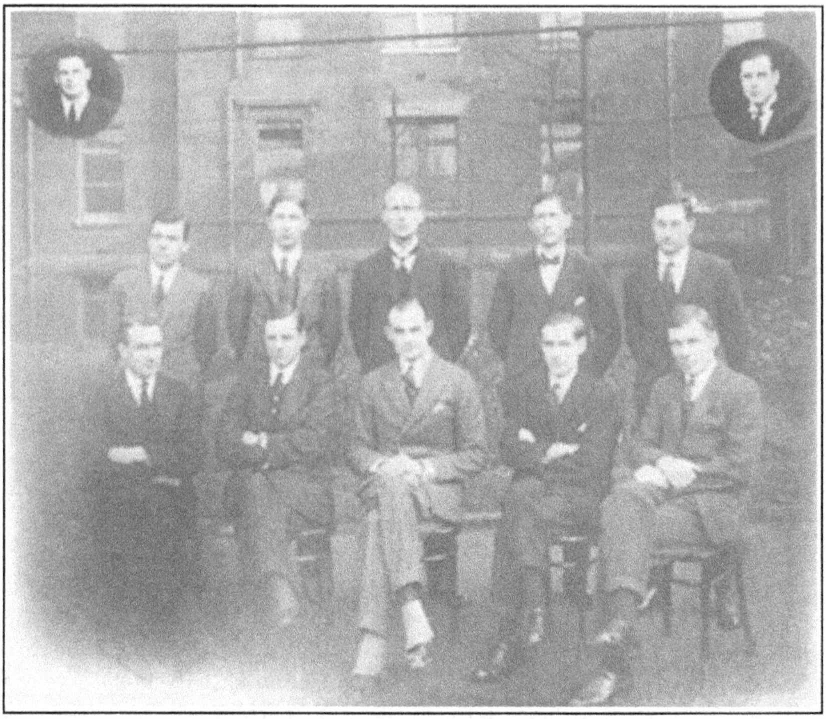

Figure 3.2: The First Assistants at The London Hospital in 1925. Bailey is in the inset in the upper right corner. McNeill Love is second from the left in the front row. In the back row are Russell Brain (later Lord Brain PRCP), Donald Hunter, the founder of occupational medicine, and in the front row is Hugh Cairns, the neurosurgeon, later Professor of Surgery at Oxford

In contrast with the Consultants who were unpaid, and the House Surgeons who received free board, lodging and beer but nothing else, the Registrars were granted a salary, though it was barely enough to live on, and certainly inadequate for the support of a wife and family. They accepted this grinding toil because of the training and experience that it afforded, and also because of the virtual certainty of a secure and lucrative career at the end of a few years. The highest prize of all was a post at one's own or, even better, at a rival London teaching hospital, but many preferred to work in a provincial city, which offered a gentler and less demanding pattern of life. Obviously, relations between four or five intensely ambitious young men caught up in this hectic existence and all competing for the same prizes gave rise to bitter rivalries and at times to hostilities and betrayals. Some dropped out of the race altogether, others no doubt became embittered and cynical, and others succumbed to illnesses.

It was while working for Sir Hugh Rigby, early in 1924, that Bailey injured his left index finger during an emergency operation for septic peritonitis. Over the next few days the infection spread rapidly into the tissue spaces of the hand and up the arm and he developed a high fever. In those pre-antibiotic days the only available treatment was surgical incision of the affected area to search for and release pus. As there was clearly no improvement Rigby operated on his young colleague, and was relieved to discover an abscess, which he opened and drained. The problem then subsided and Bailey made a complete recovery, albeit with a stiff and useless left index. (Humphries' account is different in that he says that Rigby failed to find any pus, which would in fact have made the situation worse, by encouraging spread of the infection into previously intact tissue planes. However the hospital's diagnostic index for 1924 quite clearly records 'pus evacuated - did well'.)

Bailey was advised to undergo an amputation, and to relinquish any hopes of a surgical career. The decision was agonising, but there was no point to be gained by retaining the finger, which interfered with the function of his hand. Rigby persuaded him to accept its loss, and, wisely, amputated through the end of the metacarpal bone, thus producing a shapely though somewhat narrow hand. In fact, the disability caused by this amputation is surprisingly slight, especially if it involves the non-dominant side of the body, and when he got back to work Bailey found that his operating was quite unimpaired, though he always took care to invert the index finger of his left rubber glove. In later years he even went so far as to claim that a narrow left hand was a positive advantage to a surgeon, as it could be gently insinuated into the abdominal cavity so as to feel the contents (Figure 3.3).

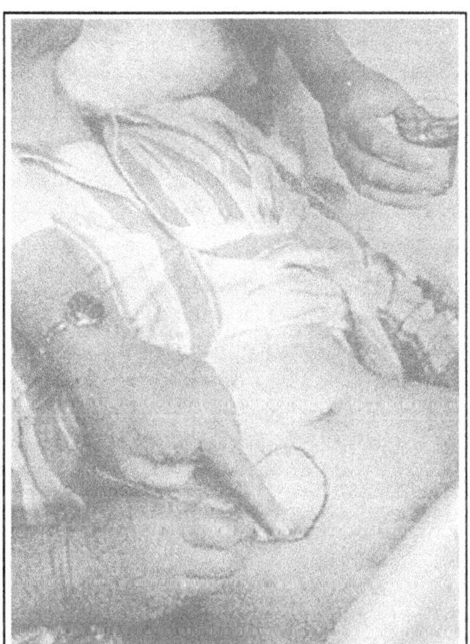

Figure 3.3: Bailey examines an abdominal mass. Note the amputated left index finger

There was an ironic sequel to this tale, in that the patient from whom Bailey's finger became infected died from peritonitis.

By the end of 1925, Bailey's accumulated experience was such that he was ready to apply for a consultant post. A vacancy arose. Mr Openshaw had died, and the post of Assistant Surgeon to The London Hospital was advertised. All the local registrars who were eligible entered the race, and there were many outside aspirants for this prize appointment. The excitement was tremendous. From dozens of hopefuls, a short list was drawn up, and on 1 November the Medical Council met to consider the applications from Messrs Ogier Ward, W. H. Ogilvie, J. D. Driberg, G. P. B. Huddy. A. C. Perry, R. J. McNeill Love, and Hamilton Bailey. The voting was as follows: Mr Driberg received 19 votes, Mr Love received 14 votes, Mr Ward received one vote, and the others none at all. The Council decided to recommend Mr Driberg to the House Committee for the vacant post.

Of these candidates, the only one not to achieve a substantial reputation in later life was Driberg. He had been awarded the Military Cross in 1916, but this apart has been described as a total nonentity. Once appointed, he made no contribution whatever to his teaching hospital. He is remembered, if at all, as having been the elder brother of the gay left wing Member of Parliament and Life Peer, Tom Driberg, of dubious reputation, whose home he shared when he eventually retired. The other applicants went on to substantial achievements, though not to the same extent as Hamilton Bailey, who had already become widely known as a teacher and author, and who received absolutely no support.

What prompted the Committee to make this incomprehensible choice? The surgical world of London was fascinated by the appointment and there was much speculation as to its reasons. It was widely hinted that Driberg owed his success to his being a Freemason, but this sort of rumour always circulated and there is nothing to suggest that it had any foundation. Appointments' committees composed of insiders tend to choose safe colleagues who will not rock the boat or disturb the peace by being inconveniently talented, and Bailey certainly did not fit this mould. From the previous record, there is every reason to suppose that he must have made some influential enemies. Deanesly was no doubt approached, and one could imagine that his comments were unhelpful. Bailey's reactions are not recorded, but those who knew him in later life all take the view that he was devastated by this rejection, which was completely unforeseen. In any event, having decided that future prospects at The London were now ruled out, he applied for and was accepted for the position of Assistant Surgeon to the Liverpool Royal infirmary. He returned to Liverpool in February 1925 and started work on 2 March.

Back to Liverpool

As Assistant Surgeon, this was his first consultant appointment. The three senior surgeons at the time were Sir Robert Kelly, Sir John Wolfenden, and Frank Jeans, whose assistant he became. The position of junior surgeon was most irksome. The senior man on the firm had complete control of all the beds and made all the decisions regarding admissions and operations. The assistant was in charge of the Out-Patient Clinics, but had no jurisdiction over whom he would treat when they were admitted. If a 'case' appeared interesting or exceptional, or coincided with the senior's professional hobby, then he would take over and the assistant would be brushed aside. Furthermore, it was entirely up to the senior man to allocate the emergency work.

When Bailey arrived, Jeans was on holiday, and for the first two months he had forty beds to himself, full control of the out-patient clinic and admissions, and supervision of the junior staff - the sort of situation which he had always sought. But at the end of this time things became difficult. To be assistant to Jeans was uniquely uncomfortable. Jeans was a witty, charming and selfish man, a bon viveur, renowned as the best after dinner speaker in Liverpool, but accustomed to passing on all emergency work, and indeed as much as possible of any other work, to his junior colleague. Furthermore, the hospital was at that time going through a difficult period from the financial point of view and all improvements, including the much needed alterations to the traditional circular wards, had been cancelled due to lack of money. Not only were the physical circumstances difficult, but, the medical staff were anxious and disillusioned and, as so often happens under these circumstances, various factions arose, each eager to preserve their own territory or if possible to take advantage of the confusion to expand into that of their neighbour.

As in the past, Bailey did his best to remain outside these disputes, and concentrate on his clinical work and teaching, and most importantly to draw together the notes he had made for *Demonstrations of Physical Signs in Clinical Surgery,* the book which he was then planning, and which was to run to 26 editions. This was a new type of textbook, directed at the young surgeon, practical, plainly written and based entirely on the type of personal experience familiar to the reader. It depended heavily on the quality of its illustrations, which were of an entirely original type. Illustrations in medical textbooks at that time were largely in the form of engravings based on a sketch by the author, laboriously copied on to copper plate and eventually reproduced in print. Because the process was so very expensive, the pictures were limited in number, and an average medical textbook of 30,000 words would probably contain fewer than five or six of them. The process was later replaced by 'photogravure', which copied the original engraving on to light-sensitive film that could be incorporated much more easily by the printer. But the scope of simple studio photography, supplying a mass of cheaply produced illustrations, whose educational value was much more than many lines of printed text, had hardly been explored. Bailey was a keen photographer (a skill learned at St Lawrence) but he needed professional help, and looked around Liverpool for a suitable photographic studio. He eventually found one managed by Vera (she detested the name and insisted on being called Veta) Gillender, the extremely pretty 18-year-old daughter of a Swedish mother and an English ship's engineer, who had just finished her training as a commercial photographer (Figure 3.4).

Veta had a vivacious, out-going personality, self confident and sociable, very pleased at her recently formed talents, and no doubt impressed by the atten

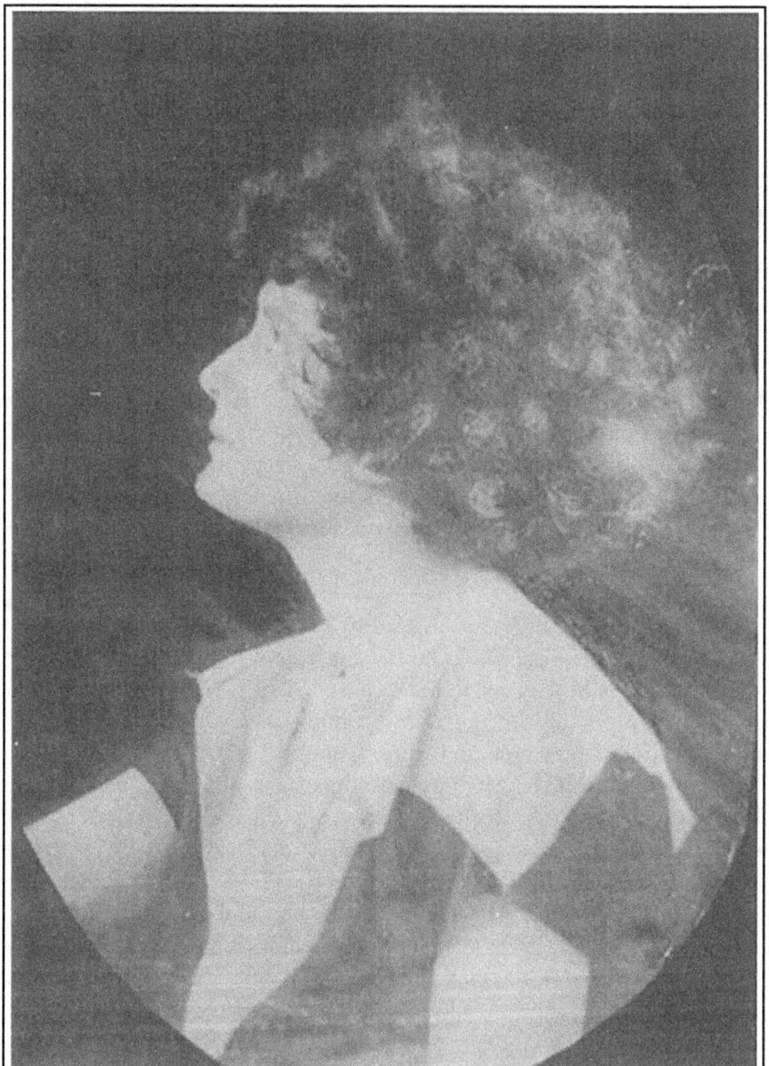

Figure 3.4: Veta Gillender, aged 18

tions of a good looking young surgeon. Bailey, in turn, was delighted to find such an agreeable and competent assistant in the work which was increasingly dominating his life. He was not sexually inexperienced (quite apart from his wartime existence, hospital life at junior level offered plenty of opportunities) and we know from later revelations that he had had at least one serious affair, but this time was different. His career seemed established, the disappointments of London had been put behind him or at least suppressed, and most of his contemporaries were married. The relationship developed from friendly professional co-operation into affectionate companionship. Veta's elder sister Dagmar, to whom Veta was very close, approved of Bailey, and encouraged their romance. He must nonetheless have been a somewhat moody and uncertain suitor, obsessed as he was with his work, preoccupied by the personal and professional problems at the Royal Infirmary, and from time to time receiving messages from Brighton following some excess on the part of his distracted mother. We have no details of their courtship, but it appears to have been fairly drawn out, as their marriage did not take place until after Bailey had left Liverpool

Over the next year his prospects at the Infirmary showed no signs of improvement. Jeans was a demanding and unsupportive colleague, and the hospital's financial and administrative problems continued. Disputes with authorities began to come to the surface, and Veta was anxious to leave Liverpool. Whether Bailey found the situation out of hand, or was asked to depart is unknown - almost certainly there was an element of both. In any event life became intolerable and he decided to take the almost unprecedented step of abandoning a consultant post at a teaching hospital post and moving to a municipal institution, where he felt that his talents would be better recognised.

Dudley Road

Dudley Road Hospital, Birmingham, though it had a high reputation for the excellent quality of its surgery and teaching, was not a particularly attractive place (Figure 3.5). Bailey took up his post there in July 1925, at a yearly salary of £700, with 180 beds shared by another surgeon, no house surgeon and most particularly no private practice, as DRH was a municipal hospital. McNeill Love came to visit him there a few months after his appointment, and noted that although he was operating seven days a week he had already accumulated hundreds of clinical photographs, mostly taken by Veta, for later inclusion in *Physical Signs*. Dr Marjorie Ball was not only his anaesthetist at Dudley Road, but also his first illustrator, making sketches of the operations as they proceeded, and supplementing Veta's photographic skills. Such was Bailey's trust in her skills that Dr Ball (later Crump) continued to draw for him long after he left Birmingham.

Hamilton and Veta were married in Birmingham on 14 January 1926. We do not know whether Dr James Bailey and Margaret were present at the occasion, but Mr and Mrs Gillender were witnesses. The young couple moved into a small 'two up two down' house at 35 Wheatsheaf Road, near to the Edgbaston reservoir, which still stands.

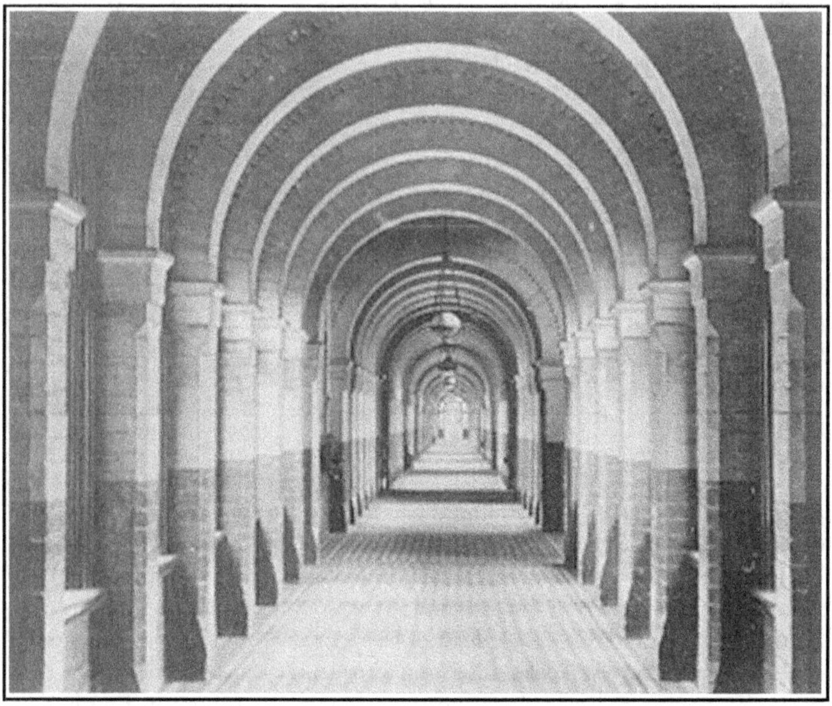

Figure 3.5: Part of Dudley Road Hospital, Birmingham, 1925 (Courtesy of the West Birmingham Health Authority).

Hamilton and Veta never came back to Liverpool. He was invited to speak at innumerable medical meetings, and must have received several offers from the Liverpool Medical Institution, but there is no record of his ever having taken them up. For Hamilton it was one of the stopping places which was so typical of his restless career, and reminded him of his past imagined failures. For Veta, always ambitious and upward moving, Liverpool represented a background which she was quite content to put behind her in her later life in the South of England. Though always obedient to the demands of Hamilton's career, she preferred to stress her Swedish origins rather than those from the mercantile North-West.

Bailey's four years at Dudley Road represented another stage in his surgical maturation. During his time there he performed 3642 operations, each faithfully set down by the Registrar in the theatre record. In most cases, the actual time of the operation is entered, and we can see that Bailey was in the theatre on a 24 hour basis. Surgery is recorded at 5.30 am and 11.30 pm every day of the week. In addition, he continued to write and to teach, and introduced a number of innovations into the practice of the hospital, including a recovery room for post-operative patients and for serious accident casualties, and a ban on the use of talcum powder for rubber gloves. Following pressure from Bailey, Dudley Road was one of the first hospitals to adopt blood transfusion, though the Management Committee only accepted it on the condition that all transfusions were given by the chief surgeon. Some of his ideas would today seem rather perverse. Thus when Carl Krebs visited his ward in 1929 he enquired why there were so many holes in the sheets, he was told that Mr Bailey always encouraged his patients to smoke a cigarette on recovering from an anaesthetic, as this assisted respiration. Quite often of course the patient would doze off again, with the inevitable result.

The first edition of *Demonstrations of Physical Signs in Clinical Surgery*, which contained over 100 photographs taken by Veta, and which was to run to 26 editions, was published in 1927. *Physical Signs* was the subject of an excoriating review in, of all places, the *London Hospital Gazette*. This further evidence of

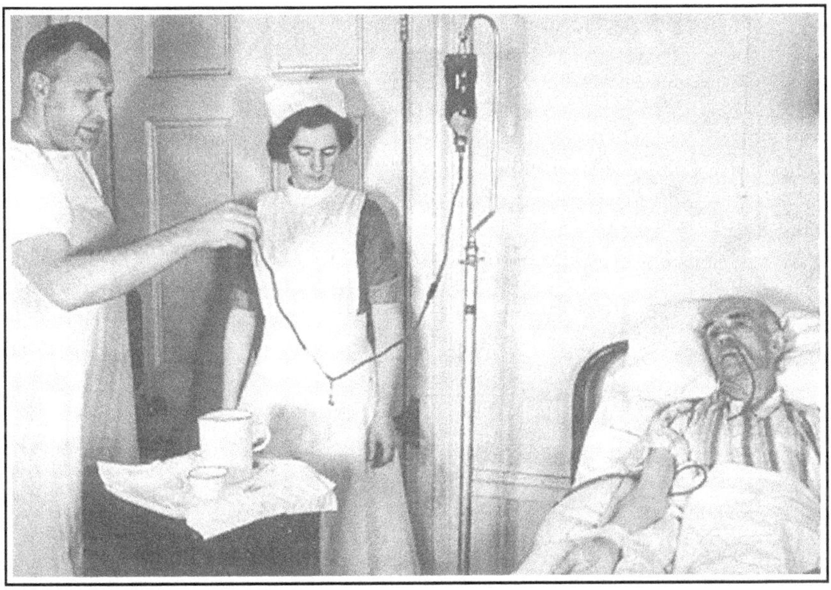

Figure 3.6: The surgeon administers a blood transfusion

antagonism originating from his teaching hospital was not lost on Bailey. Who could have written it? Although subsequent comments varied from the gentle to the enthusiastic, this particular piece, coming as it did from the alma mater to which he had given so much, and to which he had hoped one day to return, was uniquely wounding. He did not show it to Veta for two weeks.

Apart from the first edition of *Physical Signs*, 32 articles were published, and there was another book on *Branchial Cysts and other Essays*. He also started work on *Emergency Surgery*. which perhaps is the best known and most influential of all his books. Veta edited the work, helped to classify the clinical material and of course supplied the illustrations. Life at Wheatsheaf Road appears to have been settled and happy, although a miscarriage occurred shortly after they arrived.

In 1928 their son Hamilton was born, to the great delight of the Gillenders and Dr James Bailey, though Margaret's reaction is not recorded (it is likely that she was ill at the time, as this coincided with one of her many admissions to St Francis Hospital).

The four years at Dudley Road finally established Bailey's reputation as an author, and he became nationally very well known. However, there was to be no escape from political and administrative problems. As with businesses and Government departments, hospitals are hotbeds of intrigue, rivalry and gossip. The particular problem at Dudley Road was the clash between the ideologies of the

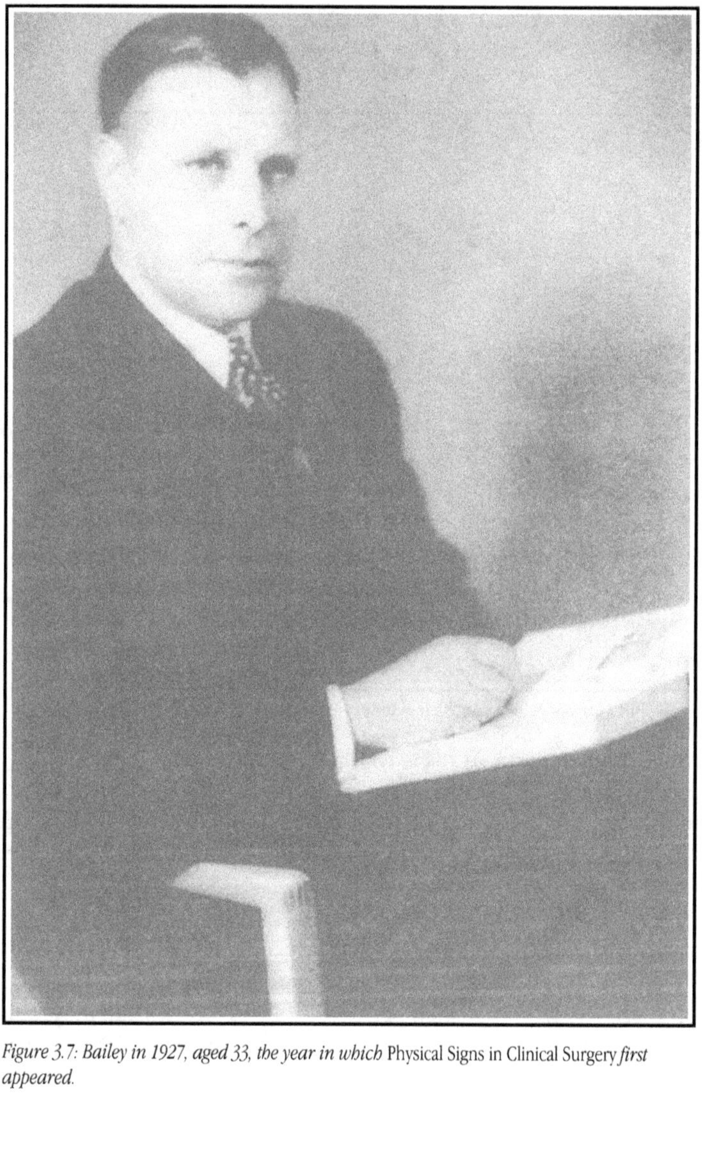

Figure 3.7: Bailey in 1927, aged 33, the year in which Physical Signs in Clinical Surgery *first appeared.*

Medical Superintendent, Frederick Ellis, who was a passionate advocate of the whole time principle, by which physicians and surgeons devoted all of their activities to the hospital, accepting a salary which they could negotiate each year using trade union procedures, and his part time colleagues, who viewed themselves as independent professionals, free to strike a bargain with any potential employer, but whose contract finally rested with the patient. In various forms, this political dialogue has continued all over the world up to the present day, and there is no sign of its ever being resolved. Bailey allied himself with the part timers. With the arrival of young Hamilton, and Veta's failure to find additional photographic work in Birmingham, his financial situation had become difficult, and he attempted to make ends meet by breaking the rules and undertaking some private practice, a move which was immediately spotted by the hospital authorities. Ellis had the support of the Hospital Guardians and the Ministry of Health, and was moreover respected as a sound and careful surgeon, whereas Bailey was an outsider and although acknowledged as a superb teacher and innovator, had acquired the reputation of being somewhat rash and hasty in the operating theatre. Nonetheless, he had allies. Many of his colleagues at Dudley Road were similarly short of money, and could not understand why those who worked in other hospitals in affluent Birmingham were allowed to receive private patients, unconstrained by the strict principles of the Superintendent, which not all of them shared, whereas they were denied this freedom. Bailey and his surgical colleagues Connell and Anderson (who was a bitter personal enemy of Frederick Ellis) went further in an attempt to legitimise the right to independent practice for all of the medical staff, but the authorities' reaction was furious, and the result was exactly the opposite of what they intended. Quite abruptly, the contracts for all part timers were terminated without consultation, and with no word of appreciation for past services. It took years to correct this injustice, which was perhaps partly responsible for the ill-feeling that persisted for a long time between the whole- and part-timers in the City of Birmingham, a view confirmed by Frederick's son Dr Hugh Ellis, himself a distinguished paediatrician.

As a result of all this fruitless conflict, Bailey was once more overtaken by restlessness and dissatisfaction. He had not quite given up hope of a teaching hospital appointment, and made enquiries in Bristol, where some of his old friends and colleagues were working at the Royal Infirmary. No post was immediately available there, but it turned out that the Bristol Homeopathic Hospital was looking for a surgeon, and negotiations began.

Bristol

Following its decline as a slave port and major trading post for the West Indies, Bristol had become the tobacco capital of Britain, dominated by the firm founded by the brothers W. D. and H. O. Wills, the manufacturers of Gold Flake, Woodbines and the small cheroots known as Wills Whiffs. The Wills family was instrumental in establishing Bristol University, and the massive Wills Tower still stands in the centre of the town. Their philanthropy extended to founding the Bruce Wills Memorial Hospital, but certain members of the family, like some of our own Royal family, became disillusioned with conventional medicine and turned to homeopathy, so that within a few years the Wills Memorial was renamed the Bristol Homeopathic Hospital. Because some influential Wills's had been successfully treated by a homeopathic physician called Bodman, the hospital was entrusted to his direction, and quite soon became the private domain of the Bodman family, who composed both the governing body and the medical staff. The senior surgeon was Mr C. Osmond Bodman, his deputy was Mr J. Harry Bodman, and anaesthetics were delivered by Dr Frank P. Bodman. Secretarial and administrative help was provided by Mrs Elisabeth, and the Misses Jane and Mildred Bodman. In June 1928 Mr C. O. Bodman decided to retire, and to everyone's astonishment, an unrelated candidate, Lieutenant Colonel Middleton West, FRCS Ed., from the Indian Medical Service, was invited to replace him, and was awarded an operating session each Friday afternoon, and every other morning at 11.00am. However, the Colonel became restless with his conditions of employment, and resigned on 19 September 1929, to take up an appointment in London. Urgent meetings of the Medical Committee, chaired as usual by Mr Bodman, and composed of his immediate family, were held on 17 October, when a Mr Adams was invited to apply but could not accept the post, and again on 16 January 1930. Unofficial feelers had already been put out to Hamilton Bailey, who had expressed some interest, and on 23 January 1930, the Secretary informed the Committee that he had once again approached Bailey to ask whether he would consider taking over the duties of Honorary Surgeon to the Hospital on a temporary basis, as this would enable him to have more knowledge of the local scene and give him an opportunity of making enquiries in the Bristol region as to the possibility of obtaining other surgical work. The Committee felt that while they would gladly welcome Mr Hamilton Bailey to the hospital, they considered that this appointment would not enough on its own to attract him to Bristol.

When these manoeuvres became known to his colleagues in Birmingham, they lost patience and asked Bailey to leave. He had probably already decided to go, but this left him no choice. On 4 January 1930 he wrote to Dr Bodman, stating that he thought the idea of accepting the appointment on a temporary basis was a good one, and that if the Committee agreed, he would plan to arrive next week, and stay for a few months, to see how it worked out. This would perhaps improve his chances with any other appointment, as he would then be resident in the district. It is quite clear from the tone of the letter that Bailey saw the post at the Homeopathic Hospital as a stepping stone to better things in Bristol. The Committee welcomed the suggestion and unanimously recommended that Mr Hamilton Bailey should be appointed temporary Honorary Surgeon to the Homeopathic Hospital. No doubt Frederick Ellis was delighted to see him depart.

By all accounts Bailey's work in Bristol was successful and appreciated. Between February 1930 and February 1931 he carried out some 500 operations at the Homeopathic Hospital, mainly of a fairly minor nature but with a heavy accent on urology, including a large number of cystoscopies. His experience in urology gained at the London was especially useful, and he set up the first urological clinic in the Bristol area (indeed when he left Bristol his services had become so essential that he was persuaded to retain his appointment as honorary urologist on a temporary basis, travelling back whenever his other commitments permitted). But although his work also extended to the Royal Mineral Water Hospital in Bath, the resources of the Homeopathic Hospital, with its limited budget, few referrals and an accent on drug treatment rather than surgery, were never going to satisfy a surgeon of Bailey's energy and aspirations. It was clear to everybody in the city that he was aiming to join the staff of the Bristol Royal Infirmary, and it was a bitter disappointment to him when he failed to secure the vacancy which occurred within a few months of his arrival. His dealings with the senior staff at the Infirmary, however, were not always tactful. Patrick Butler was a Registrar in Bristol at the time and recollected the weekly teaching sessions held in the Pathological Museum by the senior surgeon, a Mr Rendle Short, whose name reflected his choleric temper. Bailey was a regular attender at these sessions (which were really meant for students) and stood in the back row writing busily in his notepad. Short knew very well that Bailey was planning a major textbook, and would occasionally look over the rows of students to the back of the room and exclaim 'start a new paragraph now!' When, in 1932, the first edition of *A Short Practice of Surgery* by Bailey and Love appeared, there were some who made use of the unforeseen pun. But in fairness to Bailey, whatever his faults, plagiarism and failure to acknowledge primary sources were not among them. Short's name appears in all the early editions, and there is nothing to suggest that he bore any resentment for the way in which his rather unusual pupil made use of the lectures.

There is little information on Bailey's family life during this period, and it seems that Veta and young Hamilton did not accompany him on what was most likely seen as an exploratory visit, waiting for something more permanent to turn up. His address during this period was still recorded as 'Wheatsheaf Road, Edgbaston', although some letters are recorded as coming from 6 Lansdown Place, Clifton, which may have been rented rooms. But it was during this time in Bristol that *Emergency Surgery*, Bailey's third and arguably his most influential book, was published. Although Bailey had accumulated an enormous experience during these formative years, he had hesitated to record it in book form because of deference to one of his teachers at The London, Russell Howard, who had written a rather unsuccessful work entitled *Surgical Emergencies* two years before. No doubt he still felt the need not to alienate his patrons there, in case another opportunity arose to join the staff. The first volume appeared in October 1930, the second a year later when he had returned to London. In the Preface to the first edition he mentions that his wife had typed every word, had kept his case index in order and helped him to construct the composite photographs.

It is difficult to exaggerate the importance of this book or to overestimate the number of lives it must have saved. All over the world, young doctors with very little surgical training, called upon to cope with an unfamiliar emergency, used Bailey's *Emergency Surgery*, perhaps propped up against a chair in some remote primitive operating theatre, with the theatre sister or orderly reading out the steps in the operation. A typical story is that of Dr Croome from Brandon Manitoba who wrote:

> *We made the Arctic trek from Churchill, Manitoba to Edmonton Alberta in 81 days... I was the medical officer... on 13 March 1946 at Eskimo Settlement Perry River I opened the abdomen of a three year old Eskimo boy and reduced an intussusception in a native's igloo for an operating theatre. I was very grateful that I had your excellent text with me and am not ashamed to say that the successful result of the operation was due to your excellently written text rather than to any skill on my part... While crossing the Great Bear Lake my Penguin went through the ice, during which the book was completely submerged, which accounts for its present condition... I feel that you the author are entitled to it as a souvenir of the trip... .*

A battered and warped volume was enclosed with the letter (Figure 3.8).

To anyone with a knowledge of the surgical scene in Bristol in 1929, especially if the Homeopathic Hospital was involved, it was quite obvious that the Bodman family's influence was paramount. With his usual directness of purpose (or insensitivity) Bailey quite failed to recognise this, and managed, one by one, to antagonise every single member of that closely knit group. Unsurprisingly, when the next vacancy occurred at the BRI, Bailey was not appointed. The successful applicant was a man named G. R. Griffiths, who died within a few years to be succeeded by R. V. Cooke, later a Sheriff of Bristol, Vice President of the Royal College of Surgeons, a famous teacher and renowned international figure with particular expertise in the surgery of the breast and thyroid. Cooke became a close friend of Bailey, one of the few who were allowed to address him as 'Bill', and they corresponded frequently.

As soon as it became clear that he would never have the Bodmans' backing in attempts to improve his prospects, Bailey resolved to leave Bristol, and when at the end of 1930 two consultant vacancies arose at the Royal Northern Hospital in London, he immediately applied. The RNH medical committee met on 25 November and considered applications. The names included Harold Dodd (later the author of a classic work on vein surgery, with F. B. Cockett), A. J. Gardham (later senior surgeon at UCH), Harvey Jackson (who became a neurosurgeon to St Thomas's and the National Hospital Queen Square) and Thomas Holmes Sellors, whose pioneer work in cardiac surgery at The Middlesex founded the speciality in the UK, and who later was elected President of the Royal College of Surgeons. That men of this ability applied for a post at what had started as a fairly undistinguished urban voluntary hospital testifies to the position which the Royal Northern had already achieved in London surgery. The Committee recommended three names to the Board of Governors. In order of preference these were McNeill Love, Hamilton Bailey and Thomas Holmes Sellors. Love and Bailey were duly appointed.

This was a crucial moment for Bailey. He had been awarded an important post in fair competition and by the expressed wish of his colleagues, with no doubts, reservations or irregularities, and this propitious start was amply fulfilled in the years to come. Although, because of his restless energy, impatience with disagreement and often tactless and insensitive behaviour, clashes were inevitable, the Royal Northern was to be his settled professional home for the next 20 years, and it was Bailey who was mainly responsible for bringing it into the forefront of surgical teaching.

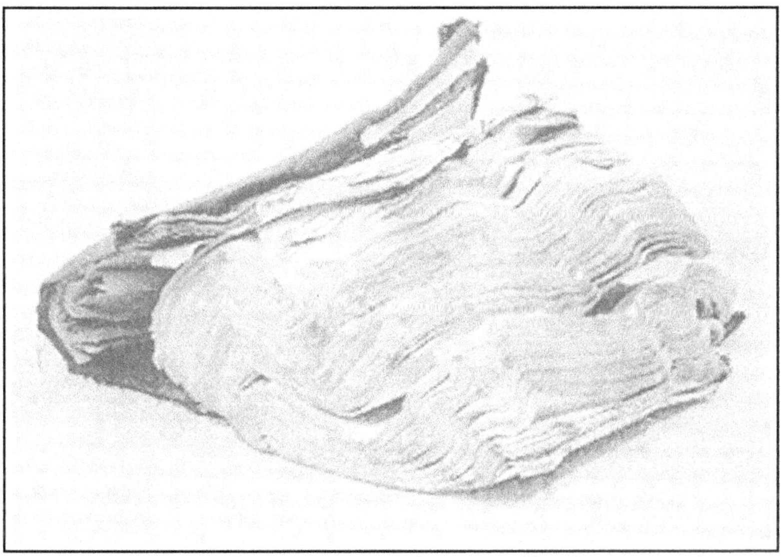

Figure 3.8: Dr Croome's copy of Emergency Surgery *which was retrieved from the Great Bear Lake*

Chapter 4

THE ROYAL NORTHERN HOSPITAL

On 15 May 1856, the following letter was received by Professor Ellis, the Dean of the Faculty of Medicine at University College London.

> *Dear Sir*
>
> *I am deeply pained at being compelled to direct your attention to the conduct of a colleague, but I feel that I should be wanting in my duty to the College were I to pass unnoticed the behaviour of Mr Statham, the Junior Assistant Surgeon, in the Theatre of the Hospital on Wednesday last 14th instant.*
>
> *While assisting Mr Footman the Assistant Medical Officer in administering chloroform to a patient on whom I was about performing a very dangerous capital operation, and who showed some litle reluctance in inhaling the vapour, Mr Statham, striking the patient in the side, said to him 'fill your bloody chest' and afterwards during the same or another operation used the same expression 'bloody' in a similar sense.*
>
> *On the same day, as I was about operating for fistula in ano, as the patient, a man, lay naked on the table, Mr Statham gave his bare buttocks a slap with the palm of the hand in an unseemly manner, exciting a laugh from the class.*
>
> *Such language and behaviour is in my opinion strongly to be deprecated when employed by an Officer connected with an educational establishment, as it sets a bad example to the students...*
>
> *Were this the only occasion in which Mr Statham had used language of a similar kind to that of which I now complain within the walls of the Hospital, I might have passed it over in silence, or contented myself with a less public mode of expressing my dissatisfaction with his conduct, but as I have had occasion before to speak to him on the same subject I feel that I have now no alternative but to bring the matter before the proper authorities of the College and to request that you will*

adopt the necessary means to prevent a repetition of such conduct, which is as prejudicial in the dignity of the College and the interests of the school as it is disagreeable to myself.

I am etc.

John Erichsen
Professor of Surgery

On 28 May of that year, following decisions by the Hospital Medical Committee, together with the Medical School Council, Sharard Freeman Statham was removed from his office and from then on was no longer assistant surgeon to University College Hospital.

Statham had been born on 17 May 1826, at Stone near Aylesbury, where his father, the Reverend Samuel Freeman Statham, was the curate. His mother, Jemima, had wealthy parents, and brought her husband a dowry of £30,000, an enormous sum in those days. Sharard was the fourth son of their marriage. In 1838 he and his brother John entered Harrow School, but he left shortly afterwards to study medicine at the recently founded secular institution of University College London. He was an outstanding student, and won the Gold Medal in his final examinations. Following qualification he worked in France and Germany, as well as nearer home, where he successfully controlled an outbreak of cholera in the small Hertfordshire town of Chesham. His many papers on gunshot injuries and fractures established his surgical reputation, and in 1851, having gained his FRCS, he was elected a Fellow of the Royal Medical and Chirurgical Society of London (now the Royal Society of Medicine) and in 1852 was elected to the consultant staff of his old teaching hospital at University College. In that respect he differed from Hamilton Bailey, but otherwise their careers were remarkably similar.

Statham was a sturdily independent character, and the records show that he was in frequent conflict with the Medical Committee and in particular with the Dean. His interest in chloroform anaesthesia, which was then a highly controversial method, produced furious arguments. He applied for leave to fight in the Crimean War (this history was to be repeated in Bailey's later life) but because of his colleagues' objections, he never left Britain. Although by all accounts a most accomplished surgeon, Statham's turbulent and resentful nature made him quite unacceptable as a team mate. The notorious 'slap on the bottom' episode in May 1856 finally brought things to a head and led to his dismissal.

For the next year or so, he conducted a successful surgical practice at No. 43 Mortimer Street. This was next to the front door of The Middlesex Hospital, and it is surprising that Statham did not seek for and obtain operating privileges there. However, the archives of the Hospital do not include his name. In 1857 Statham moved to Argyle Square near King's Cross, now one of the most notoriously sleazy and crime ridden areas of London, full of drug dealers, kerb-crawlers and dubious clubs, but at that time a respectable residential area, mainly inhabited by small shopkeepers and craftsmen. Ambitious, restless and unsatisfied by private practice, Statham determined to found a new hospital, to satisfy the growing needs of the population of North London.

A middle ground had developed between the market gardens of Middlesex, Hertfordshire and Essex and the metropolis, inhabited by the managers and clerks who worked in the centre and needed somewhere affordable to live, free from high rents and property values, but nonetheless accessible by foot or on horseback. This gave opportunities to the speculative builder, and resulted in the creation in the later years of the nineteenth century of an inner fringe of suburbs consisting of terraced houses, built to a pattern, sometimes hurriedly, and often of poor quality materials. Kentish Town and Holloway replicated, in a cheaper form, the elegant Georgian terraces of Bloomsbury and Kennington. The houses were inhabited by managers, agents, clerks, tradesmen and copywriters, who daily walked the road or took the horse-drawn bus into the City and the West End to earn a living. In turn, these people drew in the sons and daughters of agricultural workers in rural Essex and Hertfordshire, to subserve their needs, as shop assistants, manual workers and domestic servants. George and Weedon Grossmith's classic *Diary of a Nobody* gives a vivid and accurate account of the local scene.

This new bourgeoisie depended in its turn on a subservient underclass. The social contrasts at that time were dramatic. The huge and rich city of London, the financial capital of Europe and, through the British Empire, of the greater part of the developing world, contained areas of unimaginable poverty and deprivation. The young Charles Dickens wandered its streets, and immortalised his impressions. Gissing, Mayhew and others recorded for us the extraordinary vitality of the metropolis, with its mixture of prodigality and squalor. Gustav Doré came from Paris, a city where the contrast between elegance and deprivation was equally abrupt, but somehow found the predicament of the London poor more poignant and insufferable than anything he had witnessed in his country. The more affluent citizens knew little of this, and whole areas around the north and east of the capital, such as Somers Town and Hoxton, were anarchic and virtually impenetrable except by the police, who (it was said) always went in pairs. The contribution of intrepid philanthropists such as Statham reflected an awareness of historical need.

To cater for the needs of the new population and for the expanding workforce in the cattle markets and railway termini, more hospitals were needed, and this vacuum in provision occurred at the very time that Victorian philanthropy and the enthusiasm for founding 'Institutions' was at its height. The moment was ripe to start a new hospital in North London and Statham was the man to do it. Motivated by a typically Victorian combination of idealism and self interest, he leased a house at No. 11 York Road and obtained the support of Doctors G. F. Widbourne and C. P. Croft, and his brother J. L. Statham, who later was to become dental surgeon to the hospital. They met at Argyle Square on 28 July, and laid down the principles of the new hospital, which aimed to create an institution with standards equal to those of the principal London teaching hospitals. Their brief meeting produced a document which stated: 'This hospital is open to the sick poor to the extent of its means, free of letters of recommendation or any other form of admission. The management is in the hands of a Committee, chosen annually from the General body of Governors. A donation of 10 guineas or an annual subscription of 1 guinea constitutes a Governor'.

On these rather vague terms of reference, the hospital opened its doors two days later. Immediately, the patients started to arrive. During the first six months 11,718 new patients were treated, and the total number including follow-up appointments was over 28,000. Sometimes more than 300 attended in one day, including many cases of severe injury from the factories, cattle markets and railways. The treatment given must have been rather perfunctory, but the sick poor in London at that time had nowhere else to go.

For the first few months, the founders undertook all of the work, but it soon became clear that additional support was needed. A mixed committee of lay and medical members was appointed, and eventually a full medical staff. Times were not easy, and debts began to accumulate. To be a Governor appears to have been an expensive privilege, as the Governors and Medical staff made themselves responsible for clearing the debts out of their own pockets. Undeterred, the hospital continued to expand, even to the extent of hiring a nurse on a weekly wage, to care for the patients. Early in 1857 Statham persuaded the Medical Committee to enlarge the premises, so that the adjoining houses at Nos 9 and 10 York Road were acquired. It appears that the Committee were under the impression that Statham was prepared to fund the project, but in fact when they took over the accounts they were presented with a bill for some £500 which they demurred paying. To us that may seem somewhat ungenerous, in view of the immense amount of time and resource Statham had devoted to the new institute, but this kind of dispute seems to have been fairly frequent among Victorian philanthropists.

Statham died in 1858, two years after his hospital had opened. He was only 32, and the cause of death was recorded as 'phthisis' (tuberculosis) from which, unknown to his colleagues, he had been suffering for the previous two years. His total assets amounted to less than £600. He was buried at Stone, where he had been baptised and a brass plaque in the South Aisle of the church records his death with the words 'He was the Founder of the Great Northern Hospital, London'.

In spite of financial difficulties, the hospital managed to survive with the help of charitable dinners, balls and bazaars, contributions from the medical staff, committee members and local tradesmen, until 1862 when there occurred a stroke of good fortune. The Metropolitan Railway Company needed to extend their line to the North, which ran straight through the site of the Hospital, which they had to acquire. The Medical Committee submitted a claim for £5000, but this was eventually reduced to the more realistic sum of £1750. The Great Northern accepted the bid and was able to discharge its debts. After one or two temporary moves to Pentonville and the Caledonian Road, a site was eventually found in Holloway, which was bought for £7250 in 1884

There had been a move to create another hospital nearby, to accommodate the increased population, to be called the 'Central Hospital for North London'. This antagonised the medical staff of the existing Great Northern, who prevailed upon their President, the Duke of Westminster, to induce the proponents of the new scheme to unite with the Great Northern, with the new hospital to be called 'The Great Northern Central Hospital'. This was agreed, money was collected, architects appointed and a new building was finally opened by King Edward VII and Queen Alexandra on July 17 1888, with 64 beds, a large out-patient department, and a nurses' home. From there on, the newly named 'Royal Northern Hospital' rapidly achieved a major reputation, in spite of opposition from the established local general practitioners, who saw the out-patient department as a potential threat to their private practice. The *British Medical Journal* of 26 December 1891 declared 'It is believed that most of the evils which have hitherto attended the out-patients system have been met by the Great Northern scheme. Persons attempting to obtain gratuitous relief, to which their circumstances do not entitle them, have been promptly sent back to their own medical attendants'. In other words, an informal means test was in use, to ensure that charitable money only went to worthy recipients. The interests of both morality and commerce were satisfied. In 1895 the hospital's activities were so well established that it became officially recognised by the Royal Colleges as a place where medical students could be trained, and recognition came later for the training of postgraduates.

One of the most interesting features of the Royal Northern was the circular ward. This pattern, which was quite contrary to the principles laid down by Florence Nightingale, placed the nurses' station, headed by the Ward Sister, with dressing trolleys, patients' records, drug cupboards and other necessaries, housed in a vast cabinet known as 'the ambulance' at the centre of the circle, while the patients were disposed radially around the edges (Figure 4.1). This allowed the senior nursing staff to supervise and control everything that happened in the ward, and was extremely efficient. Privacy was not thought an important consideration in the case of the lower orders. The same pattern had been adopted by the Liverpool Royal Infirmary, where Bailey was later to work, but was never suggested for the more delicately minded patients in the private St David's Wing.

In the early years of this century, the Royal Northern Hospital continued to flourish, serving the needs of North London, and attracting private and municipal money, as a deserving charity. However, times were changing, and society was becoming more conscious of its debt to the underprivileged and the sick.

A mile up the hill, the smallpox hospital, later known as the Whittington, with its three wings, the Archway, St Mary's and Highgate, arose as a charitable institution, with physicians and surgeons appointed by the local authorities and the

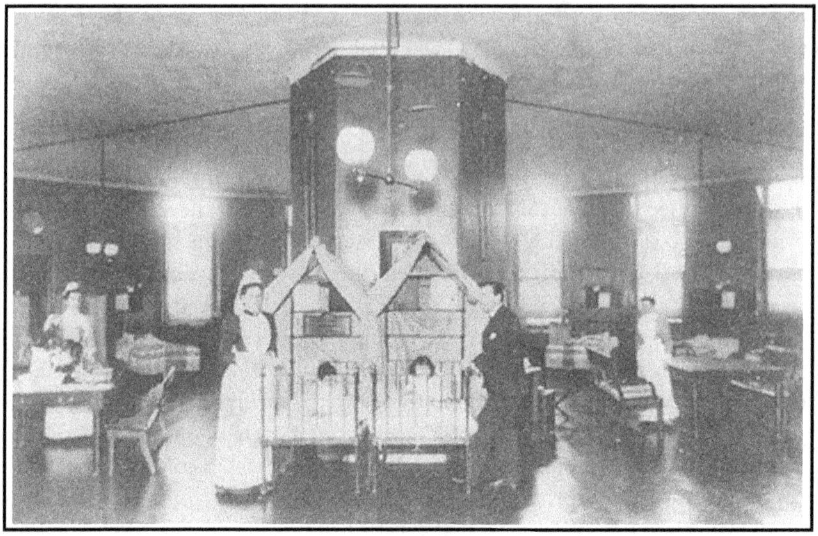

Figure 4.1: A circular ward

London County Council. This development was strengthened by the introduction in 1924 of the panel system of health insurance, by the Lloyd George government. This gave rise to antagonism between the so called Poor Law hospitals which were state funded,and the voluntary institutions which depended upon local charity, and indeed upon local wealth. The medical staff at the Whittington were salaried and appointed by the local authority, whereas those at the Northern were honorary, in that they gave their services free of charge, but gained clinical experience through the appointment, and were able to demonstrate to local practitioners that they were fit to be entrusted with private patients. The local Councillors in Islington were thus able to discharge their public consciences and their private medical needs by supporting the Royal Northern. This led to the establishment of St David's Wing, for the use of patients who could not afford the expensive private clinics of central London, but nonetheless wished to avoid the rigours of the public ward. The Marquis of Northampton, who was Chairman of the Board of Governors at the Northern, had no difficulty in gaining Royal approval for his appeal for funds to build a special pay beds block for patients of moderate means.

By 1930, the year in which Bailey was to arrive, the Royal Northern was a thriving institution, supported by local charities, exemplified by the names of the Wards, such as 'League of Roses', 'Richard Cloudesley', 'Annie Zunz', each of which represented an individual benefaction. In 1928 Lord Jellicoe, Bailey's former commander at Jutland and by now an Admiral of the Fleet, unveiled a cot in the childrens' wards which had been paid for by tinfoil collected by the 1st St Pancras Troop of Scouts and Wolf Cubs. There was a flourishing nursing school and facilities for training physiotherapists and radiographers. The Duchess of York (Queen Elizabeth the Queen Mother) opened a new maternity wing in 1932. A distinguished professional staff had been recruited. On the medical side were Geoffrey Horder (later Lord Horder and Physician to George V), Raymond Greene from the Suffolk brewing family, brother to Graham Greene the writer and Hugh Greene Director of the BBC, and a renowned expert on thyroid disease. The surgeons included Sir Lancelot Barrington Ward, W. B. Gabriel the foremost coloproctologist of the day, the urologist Kenneth Walker and of course McNeill Love, Bailey's old friend and rival from London Hospital days, with whom he was to co-operate so fruitfully in the years to come.

The hospital in 1930 presented a dignified red brick frontage to the Holloway Road (Figure 4.2). Behind this lay the ward blocks, to the north side a cylindrical building composed of superimposed circular wards, to the south a more conventional 'Nightingale' block of standard rectangular wards, which contained the operating theatres. There was a consultants' sitting room on the first floor, a Board Room for committee meetings, and on the second floor of the hospital lay the series of small cold bedrooms allocated to the junior medical staff. The outpatient department, where Bailey conducted most of his teaching, was at the extreme south end of the hospital, to which was attached the St David's Wing for private patients. This wing had a flat roof, towards which visitors were rather optimistically directed by signposts indicating the 'Sun Lounge'. It would have been difficult to acquire much of a tan in the Islington the 1930's, given the few ultraviolet rays which penetrated the deep fog of the capital.

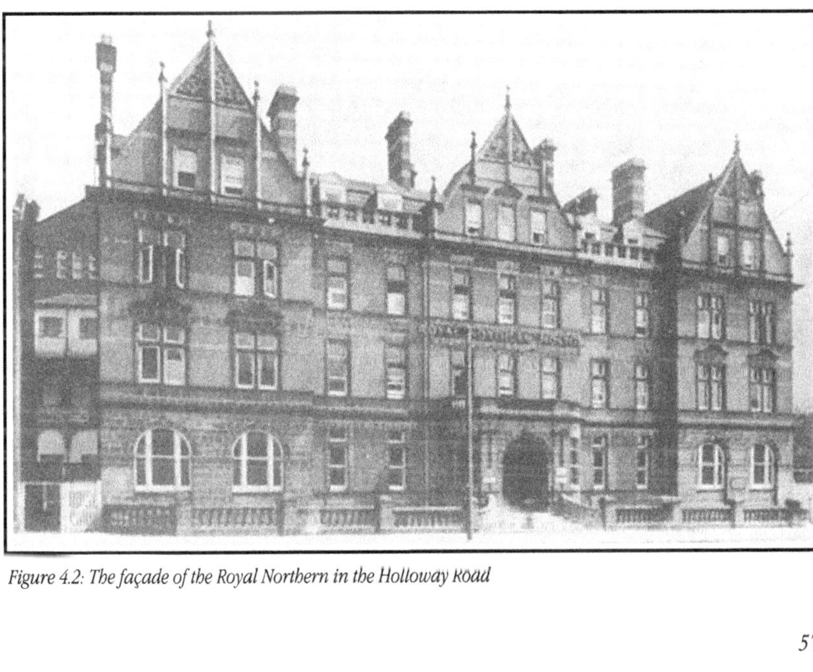

Figure 4.2: The façade of the Royal Northern in the Holloway Road

The events of the Second World War are described in Chapter 6. The Royal Northern Hospital continued to flourish for many years after Bailey's death, and attracted a distinguished medical staff, most of whom held parallel appointments at the major teaching hospitals. However, with the reorganisation of health services in London in the 1970s, involving the closure of many hospitals, the decision was made to site the main District Hospital for Islington on the Whittington site, on Highgate Hill. This was bitterly opposed by the medical staff of the Royal Northern at the time, but the situation was resolved by making a series of joint appointments, so that the physicians and surgeons at the Whittington also had clinical facilities at the Royal Northern. As the Royal Northern was progressively depleted of funds, morale fell off, the casualty department and the nursing school disappeared, and all services were transferred to the Whittington. The hospital finally closed in 1992, thus bringing to an end 140 years of public service, spanning five reigns, two world wars and several radical revisions of health care. The shell of the hospital still exists, and the boarded up façade can be seen in the Holloway Road. An attempt was made to preserve the name, by giving it to the new wing at the Whittington, but the prefix 'Royal' cannot legally be transferred, so that the facility is called 'The Great Northern Wing' (Figure 4.3). This was the original name of the hospital, so that historical honour is satisfied. However, the building is derelict, and the Hamilton Bailey archive had to be rescued from within a pile of dust and debris, before its transfer to the archives of the Royal London Hospital.

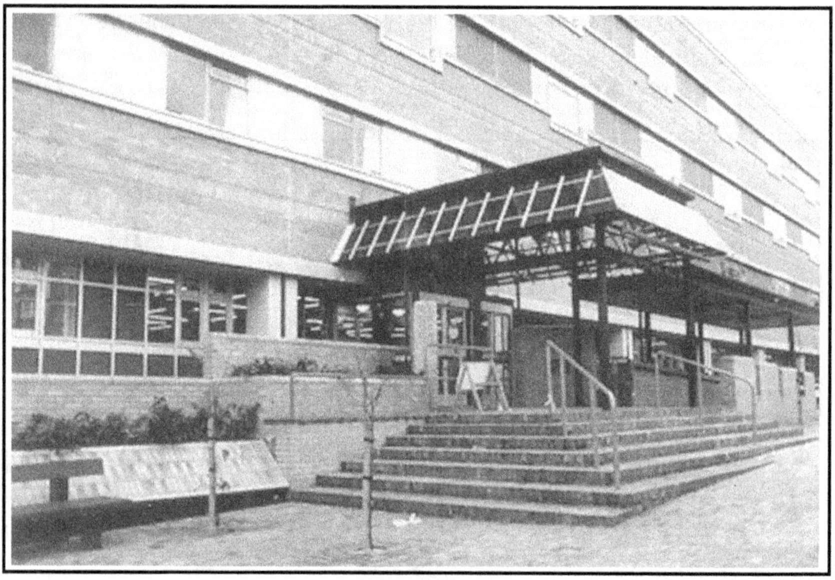

Figure 4.3: The Great Northern Building at the Whittington Hospital

Chapter 5

FAIRLAWN

The Royal Northern was the hospital to which Hamilton Bailey was appointed in 1930, and which was to be his workplace for the next 20 years. The post was charitable, in that the honorary consultants received no salary. It was philanthropic, in that it provided a service for many thousands of sick people who had little income and no capital. It was at the same professionally useful, in that it gave the consultants access to a broad range of disease, which they could use for their personal education and for inclusion in articles and books. Finally, it was lucrative, in that the local general practitioners, almost all of whom had some proportion of private practice, preferred to send their paying patients to those consultants whom they knew to be accessible and reliable in the charitable sphere. A past president of the American College of Surgeons is on record as saying that the necessary qualities for the establishment of a successful practice are 'availability, affability and ability', in that order. Bailey fulfilled all these criteria. He was seemingly tireless, always accessible, and the meticulous and prompt way in which he replied to every clinical approach made him an immediate success with the general practitioners of North London, who were a group of astute and competent doctors. That his operations did not always lead to a cure was a consideration that applied to all of his colleagues, and there were no league tables by which performances could be compared.

On taking up his new appointment, Bailey immediately set to work with his usual energy and enthusiasm. The Medical Committee arranged a rota for the surgeons' emergency responsibilities, so that three out of the five Honorary Staff were always available, and it was agreed that Bailey should be first on call on Fridays (the least popular day of the week), second on Tuesdays and third on Thursdays. The Royal Northern had never had an expert in urology, and part of his duties was to act as their first urologist. He set up a cystoscopy clinic, in space unwillingly yielded by the fracture department, which he personally manned until the appointment of Valentine Swain, who relieved him of much of the work.

Bailey's arrival at the Royal Northern made a huge impact on both the man and the institution. The appointment gave him back the self confidence that had been badly shaken in Birmingham, Wolverhampton, and Bristol, and by his rejection by the London teaching hospitals. The acquisition of a respected position where his talents were recognised, where there was no need to impress, and in which he was in complete command of his life provided a base of stability which gave him the freedom to that which he loved doing and was best at, namely writing and teaching. At the same time, from being a well regarded but not especially different urban voluntary hospital, the Royal Northern became to be seen as a 'centre of excellence', purely because it was the hospital in which the famous author worked. The combination of Bailey and the Northern produced a remarkable increase in British surgical prestige. The appearance in 1939 of the *Royal Northern Textbook of Operative Surgery* was an example, but this was overshadowed by the huge output of Bailey's books, which occurred throughout the 1930s.

Brighton again

When Bailey and Veta first moved to London in 1930, Dr James Bailey, relieved by his son's determination to settle down to a metropolitan career, bought the couple a small semidetached house in Hendon. He was able to do this because the fluctuating circumstances in Brighton had finally changed in his favour. Brighton had profited greatly from the 1914-18 war. The many German waiters and cooks employed in the hotels left hurriedly at the declaration but were replaced by Belgian and French refugees, and the population expanded by 30,000. The local Chamber of Commerce anticipated an upsurge in demand following the destruction of their competitors in Boulogne, Ostend and Deauville but, however, 1918 was followed by a depression. The aquarium was £23 000 in debt, the municipal orchestra had to be disbanded, and there was a rise in poverty and unemployment. Many Welsh miners migrated to southern towns in search of work which they never found. The General Strike of 1926 produced riots among the railwaymen, culminating in the famous 'Battle of Lewes Road' in which strikers attempting to halt rail and bus transport were confronted by a strange alliance of police, local bourgeoisie and retired cavalry officers, and were eventually driven back without being given the opportunity of presenting their petition. The strikers must have passed Dr Bailey's window. There is no record of his reaction, but his practice certainly suffered during these years.

The 1920s gave Brighton a renaissance. This was the era of Sir Harry Preston, the owner of the racecourse and of two major hotels, a famous entrepreneur who devoted much energy and money to his favoured city and gave his name to its largest pleasure park. Preston Park is still a pleasant place for local people to walk around in. Tourists never go there. It was Harry Preston who stage-managed the 'Fête de France' (to this day, Brighton has close links to France and receives hundreds of French students in its language schools), and also, more importantly, cleared the slums along Carlton Hill and Sussex Street, at the same time creating new garden suburbs in the Downs, around Hangleton and Hollingbury. The electrification of the London and Brighton Railway in 1933 was the final development in this success story, which finally established the town's prosperity. We can still see the two triumphant concrete pillars set up on the London Road, below Pyecombe Down, proudly welcoming the visitor into the County Borough.

This improvement in Brighton's economy had its effect on Dr Bailey's prosperity. He moved out of Rugby Road into Brunswick Square on the Hove sea front, and his practice became more and more associated with staid and prosperous Hove rather than feckless Brighton, whose citizens often neglected to pay their doctors' bills. At the same time, his domestic problems became worse, as Margaret's periods of illness recurred, and she spent progressively longer periods locked up in St Francis' Hospital. He came to rely on his sister-in-law Edith, and also upon Veta, whom he had always liked but who had never achieved any sort of relationship with her volatile and explosive mother-in-law. Dr Bailey seldom came to London, but Veta and young Hamilton often visited him in Brighton at weekends.

Fairlawn

Hamilton and Veta were grateful for Dr Bailey's generosity in helping to establish themselves in London, but the Hendon house quickly became inadequate, and they moved to Courtland Avenue, Mill Hill, near to the famous school of that name to which young Hamilton had been entered, while Bailey took on consulting rooms at 35 Harley Street. Veta became pregnant again in 1933, but the pregnancy had to be terminated because of toxaemia. In 1934, as the practice improved and money started to come in, they were able to buy 'Fairlawn', an imposing house with four acres of garden, overlooking Totteridge Common, and to employ maidservants, a nurse for young Hamilton, and a chauffeur. Additional space was required to accommodate the number of secretaries which he needed to conduct the expanding load of clinical and literary work (Figures 5.1 and 5.2). Fairlawn is still there, and is quite magnificent, with its curved portico and sweeping lawns. Since the Baileys, it has had a number of occupants, and its present owner is a Mr Ivens, the man who introduced the telephone answering machine into Britain, and has prospered on the proceeds of this benificent piece of foresight.

Sadly, Dr James Bailey never saw his son's new dwelling, which would have made him very proud. On 3 December 1933, while sitting in his Hove surgery receiving patients, he died from a massive pulmonary embolus. Margaret's death some years earlier in St Francis Hospital is unrecorded.

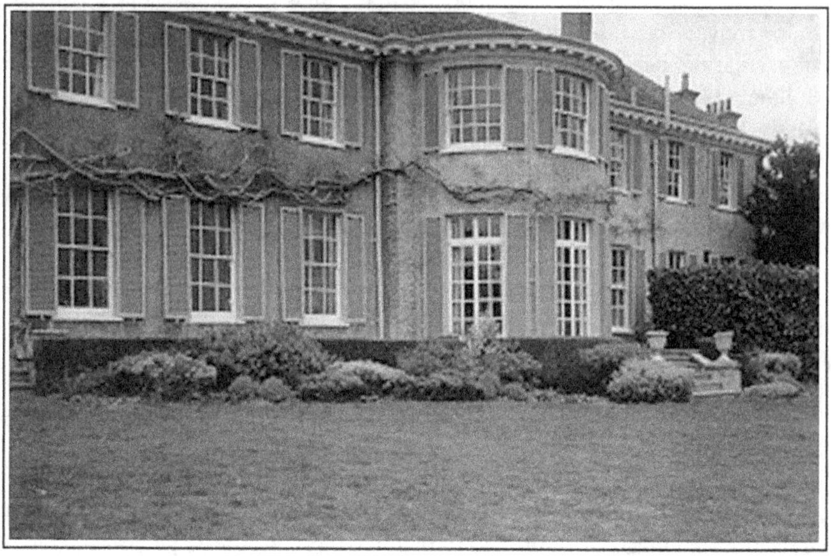

Figure 5.1: Fairlawn

Once settled in at Fairlawn, Hamilton and Veta started to develop a social life, and to entertain hospital colleagues and local general practitioners at evening receptions and dinner parties, always, however, making clear that there was a very definite end to the gathering, because of Hamilton's commitments to his books, and to his incessant round of operating lists, which started early in the morning. Dr James Thomson recollects clearly being invited to Fairlawn by Hamilton and Veta on several occasions, and remembers the generosity of the fare provided. It was clear to all, however, that these occasions always had a professional purpose, rather than being purely friendly and social. For example, there was never an exchange of children.

Guests at the Bailey household were sometimes surprised by the type of the hospitality on offer, particularly if they had not had the opportunity of meeting their host the previous evening, and were unaware of the pattern of his work. A day at Fairlawn was a fairly vigorous experience. Bailey usually slept in a small converted summerhouse overlooking the swimming pool, and got up at 5:30 am for a cold plunge. Young Hamilton was expected to join in this exercise, and the invitation was extended to anyone who happened to be staying. This was often the only time when Bailey could be approached by a visitor needing advice or help but, needless to say, the opportunity was not always taken up. After his swim, he would take a shower or bath, rub himself down with cologne and return to the house for breakfast at 7.30, where Veta would have made certain that the essential items, the gold cigarette case, cigarette lighter and pencil on the end of a chain, were in place. In the early years he drove himself to work, but later acquired a specially built Rolls Royce, which the chauffeur would bring up to the front door at 8.00 am precisely. This remarkable vehicle, which became quite famous, was divided into a small front area for the driver and a capacious rear compartment which accomodated Bailey, one or more secretaries, any visitor who happened to be there and, most notably, the Dictaphone, to which he addressed most of his conversation. The Dictaphone was a machine approaching the size of a baby grand piano, incorporating a speaking tube and a battery charged electric motor which drove a rotating wax cylinder on to which the dictation was etched by a metal stylus and recorded for eventual transcription by the secretary. The Dictaphone was supposed to be quite silent, but sometimes did not live up to its manufacturers' claims, and an important clinical message was interrrupted by the groans and clanks of an unoiled armature. But no other British surgeon was aware that such technology was available and to have seized upon this advance was the 1930 equivalent of discovering computerised word processing and e-mail, many years ahead of the competition.

In his impressive carriage, Bailey would progress slowly down Highgate Hill, dictating all the time, and arrive at the Royal Northern Hospital. The car would deposit him at the front entrance in the Holloway Road, and then be parked by the chauffeur in a side street, leaving the secretary to sort out the previous day's work. At lunch time the chauffeur would take the secretary home, collect a new wax cylinder and rejoin Bailey wherever he happened to be.

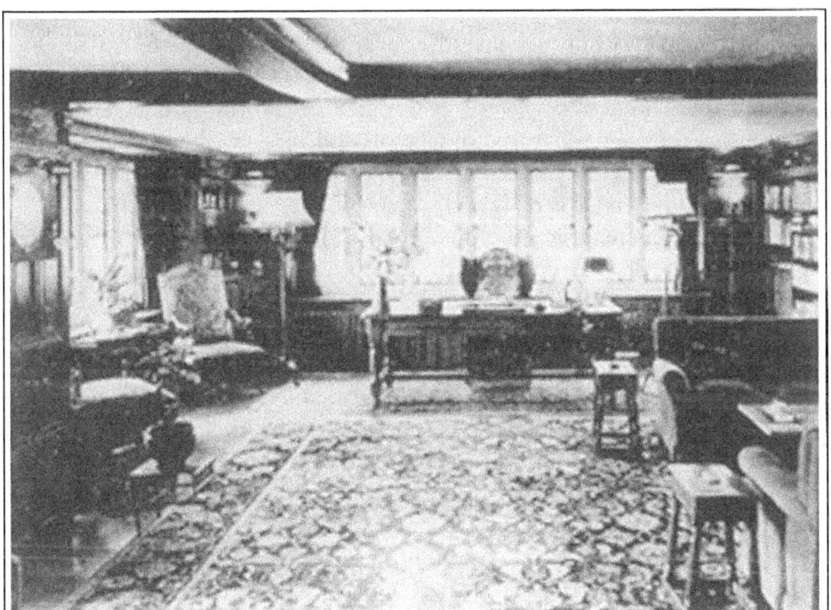

Figure 5.2: The study at Fairlawn

The Ward Round

Passing through the front door, Bailey's hat, coat and stick would be taken by a porter. Upstairs in League of Roses Ward, he would be greeted by the head nurse, always known as Sister, attended by her Staff Nurses and a small group of student nurses (probationers) standing on his right. On the left, there would be his surgical registrar, two housemen, and a group of medical students who in spite of being often reminded of their good fortune in having such a renowned teacher, for the most part had their minds on other things. As the years went on, and the books became world famous, more and more young doctors from overseas would attend these rounds. Bailey's visit was a round in the literal sense, because of the circular design of the wards at the Royal Northern. He would pause briefly at each bed, draw down the bedclothes, make a quick and decisive examination, issue instructions and pass on. Apart from a brief greeting he did not as a rule talk directly to his patients and only occasionally answered their questions. The Sister and nurses would follow him attentively, noting down his words and recording the doctor's orders. It was recognised and acknowledged that the Chief was giving his services free, and that every patient should be grateful for his attention and presence. Naturally, some of the patients 'did well', and some of them 'did badly'. To do well was to get out of hospital within two or three weeks, and to do badly was to linger on or to die. Although the nurses and students must have noticed that patients operated upon by one surgeon did rather better than those treated by another, the obvious conclusion that the first surgeon was better than the second, was never voiced, and no suggestion was ever made that the system could be improved. It was recognised that some surgeons were bold, in that they were prepared to take on difficult and complex cases which were almost bound to do badly. The fact that the heroism involved the patient's life rather more than that of the surgeon was conveniently overlooked. The system was hierarchical, and the mixture of frustration and sycophancy which attended the practice of a consultant in the earlier years of this century is almost unimaginable, until one attends a Court of Law, and observes the attitude of the barristers and officials towards the presiding Judge. Nonetheless, in the circumstances of the time, it was not the worst alternative.

At the end of the round the group would retire to Sister's sitting room, where Bailey would find a small lace covered tray at his side, with his cup, silver milk jug and plate of biscuits. It was the duty of Sister's Maid to provide this little service. Sister's Maid, dressed in cap and apron, was often an ex-patient who, having been rescued from some prolonged illness on the ward, found herself with no home to return to, and was grateful to be selected for this humble but secure livelihood. Bailey would sit down on one side of the gas fire, with the Sister on the other, and the junior medical staff either standing or seated around him. The staff nurses were allowed to attend this gathering, but the probationers were excluded. Each case folder was taken up, the morning's decisions confirmed with Sister, and the operating list for the next day arranged accordingly. The whole process of ward round, meeting and discussion would take perhaps two hours, unless students from the London Hospital were present, in which case it was prolonged because of the demands of teaching and answering questions. Walking back down the stairs to the entrance in the Holloway Road, accompanied by houseman and registrar, Bailey would find the Rolls Royce waiting for him, with the Dictaphone safely installed in the rear compartment. Ushered in by the chauffeur, Bailey would immediately start up the machine and begin recording on to the wax cylinder letters to general practitioners and colleagues, random surgical thoughts, case histories, and notes for Veta in respect of the book he was currently writing. In this dignified way, he would proceed to the next appointment, either in Harley Street, or to one of his many other hospitals or a house call.

Upstairs in League of Roses Ward, once the medical team had left, a second round took place, at which the Sister and her staff nurses would visit each bed to explain what the doctors had meant and what decisions had been made, and quite often to alleviate the uncertainty and distress that had been occasioned by their presence.

The House Call

Dr James Thomson recalls that when he arrived from Aberdeen in 1932, to take up his uncle's practice in North London, he made tactful enquries about the local surgeons, and was quickly informed that the best man in the neighbourhood was Hamilton Bailey, who was always available, either to visit a patient at his or her home or to arrange an admission. Whatever the nature of the encounter, an accurately typed letter would arrived by first post the following day. This quite exceptional service was provided by no other surgeon in the neighbourhood.

Dr Edward Baron was a respected General Practitioner in Tottenham. He sent all of his surgical patients to Bailey and his confidence was such that when members of his family became ill he had no hesitation in confiding them to Bailey's care. The eminent gastro-enterologist and medical historian Hugh Baron recollects that at the age of twelve he received his appendix from Bailey in a small bottle, which for many years he kept on his mantelpiece. Marriage brought about a reorganisation of family possessions, and his new wife saw little attraction in this trophy, which went its way. If it were possible to retrieve it, it would be interesting to test Bailey's diagnostic ability by submitting the specimen to examination by a modern pathologist. Preserved in formalin the signs of acute inflammation would still be there, if they were ever present.

In the 1930s, when Lloyd George's panel system was still developing, and the Welfare State had not been thought of, relations between general practitioners and consultants were subject to a rigid system of etiquette and protocol, designed to protect ownership of the patient. The patient 'belonged' to the GP, so that if a second opinion was called for it was always at his (there were virtually no female doctors in the neighbourhood at that time) request. Clearly, it quite often happened that a patient felt the need of a second opinion, perhaps because of loss of confidence in his doctor, in which case he would ask his GP to provide one. The experienced GP would anticipate this, and suggest calling in an expert before the suggestion was made, always with the proviso that the patient must agree to pay. Sometimes of course a GP might not see the need do this, in which case he would invite the patient to choose between accepting his advice or seeking another doctor. In the poorer districts around the Royal Northern this situation practically never arose.

At that time most consultations took place in the patient's home, in contrast to what happens today, when we rely on instrumentation and laboratory tests to supplement simple listening and physical examination. The domiciliary visit followed a well understood ritual, with due regard to etiquette. The GP would always be the first to arrive, and when the consultant appeared an introduction would take place in the front parlour, a room seldom opened except on Christmas day, and for weddings and funerals. The GP would always take care to step ahead into the sick room, in order to introduce the consultant, and make sure that the patient was not alarmed by the sudden incursion of a stranger. Both doctors would then sit down to listen to the history. The consultant would examine the patient, carefully observed by the GP. The GP would explain to the family that the consultant wished to wash his hands. A clean towel would have been made available in some adjoining area (kitchen or scullery) to which the doctors would retire for a muttered conversation. They would then re-enter the room, the GP going first, who would say to the family (for example) 'Mr Bailey and I have considered your son's problem, and are totally agreed as to what should be done. I would like you now to hear what Mr Bailey says'. The consultant would then state his diagnosis and proposed treatment which, in Bailey's case, might well comprise immediate admission to hospital for an operation. The GP would concur. At no time in this process would the consultant be left alone with the patient. When the visit was over, the GP would be the last to leave the house.

It was almost impossible to reject this kind of doubly reinforced advice, which not only carried the stamp of authority, but also had also been paid for. Obviously, the message was not always correct. There was no point of reference, in the sense that imaging and laboratory tests were not available, and the whole system depended upon informed experience and guesswork. But it was, in the present sense of the term, 'client sensitive', in that general practitioners were quick to recognize those surgeons who, whatever the outcome of the case, gave them a prompt service which sustained their practice, in contrast to those who, however skilled and well intentioned, did not satisfy the patient. Bailey succeeded admirably in this. He was not always right, and his treatments did not always work, but he was quick, decisive, and very supportive of the referring doctor. Moreover, he was always available. If his rather brusque manner upset a member of the family, the GP was always there to explain that busy and eminent surgeons did not have the time to waste on politeness.

Private Practice

Bailey's earnings from private practice during his first year at the Royal Northern amounted to £300, but this quickly expanded and 1931 brought in £1800, which was a very respectable sum at the time. He took consulting rooms at 35 Harley Street and later moved to larger premises at No. 123, which were decorated by one of his patients, a marine artist, in lieu of a fee. He found a new photographer, Mr T. A. Nicholson, an employee of the Topical Press Agency, whom he equipped and set up in rooms in Upper Harley Street, thus relieving Veta of the burden of illustrations and releasing her for her more responsible editorial work. Nicholson's first encounter with Bailey had been rather daunting. A modest and retiring man, he had been a specialist in depicting railways, and had never been in an operating theatre. Bailey invited him to take some photographs of a thyroid operation. Having positioned and focused his camera, he was asked 'are you ready?', whereupon Bailey took up a large knife with which he appeared to slice off the patient's head. In fact the incision was only skin deep, but at that time Nicholson's knowledge of anatomy was equally superficial. Thinking that he had somehow been enticed to witness a murder, he turned pale, his knees gave way and he sank to the floor. Recovering from this experience, he learned fast, and soon found work from the many other medical authors in and around the Harley Street area. Bailey persuaded the Governors at the Royal Northern to established a photographic department and to put Nicholson in charge. He was later joined by a partner, a Mr L. T. Clifford, who produced motion pictures, which were enormously successful at lectures and meetings, especially in America. These films were always very closely monitored and supervised by the surgeon.

Bailey did not make much use of the St David's Wing for his private patients, but preferred the St Vincent's Clinic, a small Catholic nursing home in the Notting Hill area. Although not in the least religious, he seems to have developed a close affinity with the nuns and gained their affection and confidence. St Vincent's was always short of money, and quite often Bailey would forego his fee so as to provide a needed piece of equipment for Sister Pauline, who as well as running the operating theare was a qualified radiographer. He established a follow up clinic for those who could not afford fees, which prompted one of the Irish sisters to say: 'he had a strong weakness for helping those not blessed by a liberal share of wordly goods'. Dennis Dooley, an inspector of anatomy, a Latin scholar whose wife worked at St Vincent's, and who sat on the governing body, was of great help to Bailey in his charitable work for the home, and in subsequent troubles.

Bailey was conspicuously unworldly. He took no interest in medical politics, whether local or national, seldom attended committee meetings at the Royal

Northern, and unlike his old colleague and fellow author McNeill Love, was never elected to the Court or the Council of the Royal College of Surgeons. There was an underlying and largely unvoiced element of envy and distrust between Bailey and the conventional surgical establishment, who found it difficult to accept that someone so different from themselves should have acquired a worldwide reputation as a teacher and author. Although he seemed to ignore and brush off this lack of acceptance, it was deeply felt and deeply resented, as became clear later.

In several important respects Bailey's career pattern was quite different from that of the average successful London surgeon in the 1930s. For example, he was not particularly interested in money, and his fees were always modest. Veta kept the accounts, and was frequently exasperated by her husband's failure to record a particular patient whom he had been able to help get over a difficult clinical problem, but whose name, or at which address the private consultation had taken place, he was unable to remember. Bailey never collected bad debts. If someone forgot to pay him, he would forget that also. This caused Veta much anxiety because, although she was prepared to work at all hours to sustain his principles, in the last resort the financial returns from her husband's practice were her only means of future security. Her contribution to the practice was crucial. Her initial training as a photographer was one of the most important factors in the initial success of the textbooks, but she went further than this. She had innate managerial skills, and her unique knowledge of Bailey's approach to surgery, gained from innumerable pictures and revisions of chapters enabled her to respond to telephone calls from worried patients and their families, from GP's, junior surgeons and nurses, all of which she parried effectively, in defence of her husband. This is not to say that she betrayed the patients' interests. She knew very well that if she misinterpreted the urgency of the message, Bailey would be furious. Nonetheless, house surgeons and registrars at the time record that, finding themselves at a loss with an acute clinical problem they would telephone the house, and that Mrs Bailey would tell them what to do, by referring to the exact page number of the appropriate latest edition of the textbook.

The Outpatient Department

The activity in which Bailey took particular pride was his Outpatient Clinic at the Northern, managed by the formidable Sister Webb. Here he could have access to a large range of patients, satisfy his fascination with physical abnormalities, teach an admiring audience of post-graduates, and record the results in his books. There were two routes of access into the Outpatient Department, one of which was a back door entry leading directly into the consulting room, the other involving a walk through the waiting area, so that all the anxious people on the benches could see the exact time of arrival of the great man whose name was written over the door. Most of his colleagues preferred the back route, but Patricia Robin records that Bailey always made it a point of honour to come in through the same door as his patients, confident as he was that if he was late it was for a good reason. Each patient was brought into the consulting room by Sister Webb, and Bailey would take a brief history, to which he often did not listen very carefully, rather hastening to the part of the consultation which really interested him, which was to elicit the physical findings. These were carefully charted, demonstrated to the audience of students and postgraduates and, if thought useful for publication, photographed. Questions of privacy and modesty did not arise (Figure 5.3).

During the interview, a nervous or timorous patient would tend to back away from Bailey's desk, which meant that he had to follow them by edging his chair across the room. This rather undiginified pas de deux came to exasperate Bailey, who eventually solved the problem by chaining the patient's chair to the table leg. Leslie Le Quesne reports as follows:

> *During the winter of 1946-47 I was HS at St Mark's, working for Cliff Naunton Morgan and Ossie Lloyd Davies. At that time I was studying for my final FRCS. My free afternoon coincided with Hamilton Bailey's outpatient clinic at the Royal Northern Hospital. I attended the clinic regularly over a period of about three*

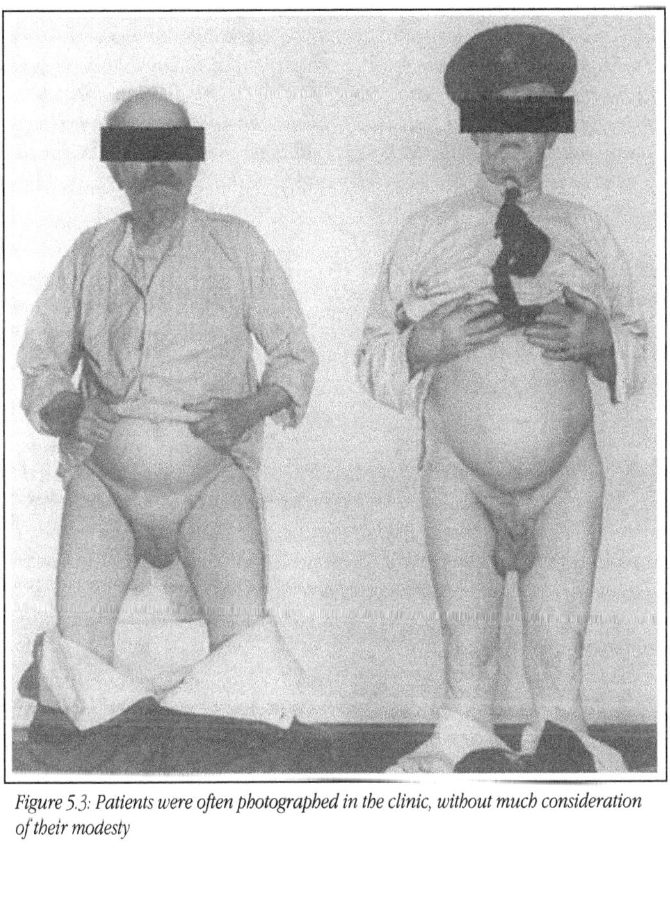

Figure 5.3: Patients were often photographed in the clinic, without much consideration of their modesty

months. The clinic was well known to people working for the final FRCS and I recall that there were always 2-3 postgraduates, usually Australian, at the clinic as well as myself. Those were of course the days when considerable numbers of Australians came over to the UK to obtain the English FRCS.

I cannot clearly remember the room in which the clinic was held, but I have a very clear idea of HB himself. He was a big man, tall and broad shouldered, with a large head, with his greying hair cut 'en brosse' (Figure 5.4) - essentially what we would now call a crew cut. He wore rubber gloves throughout the clinic with the finger process corresponding to the missing digit in his right hand (I think) being inverted. He was undoubtedly rather an intimidating figure, as he sat, towards the middle of the room at a small table with his chair, notes etc. close up to the right hand end of the table. The patient's chair was close up the right hand edge of the table, anchored to the table by a chain joining one of the chair legs to one of the legs of the table.

The patients were shown in by the Sister in charge of the clinic, sat down and HB took a brief history. If I remember correctly they were all undressed, wearing a short dressing gown. This was certainly the case with women complaining of a lump in the breast, who came in stripped to the waist but wearing a loose dressing gown. After taking a brief history, HB would part the patient's gown and palpate the breast, as the woman sat there in the middle of the room. I well remember an occasion when the patient had an obviously advanced carcinoma of the breast: as he sat there palpating the lump said to the patient 'Oh dear Oh dear, you know that you have left it too late, don't you?' Not surprisingly the patient burst into tears, whereupon HB called out 'Sister, I don't know what's wrong with the patients today. Take her away, Sister'. After all these years I cannot swear to it that these were his exact words but I clearly remember that his remarks were brief and essentially in such terms.

At that time HB was very interested in the surgical treatment of tuberculous cervical adenitis, then a common condition. He was very keen on the wide excision of the diseased nodes, through a long incision which was left open, to heal by granulation. He wrote a number of papers about this in the British Journal of Surgery *and no doubt partly as a consequence of this many patients were referred to his clinic. I remember him being very fascinated by a patient with a collar stud abscess pointing low down in the neck, between the two heads of the sternomastoid, with the result that cross fluctuation could be clavicle. He was so intrigued by this that he called over a physician who was seeing patients in a neighbouring room. I cannot recall his name (it was I think double barrelled) but I remember that he was reserved, precise, rather aloof, the exact antithesis of HB. Clearly the anatomical peculiarity of the abscess was of no interest to him, and as he went back to his clinic I heard him muttering to his house physician that HB was still at the stage of collecting birds eggs.*

It would be unfair to HB to give the impression that these two stories give a balanced picture of him, though they certainly reflect one aspect of his character. He was not only physically large, but in many ways larger than life. In his outpatients every week he saw a large number of patients with a wide range of conditions, with a wealth of clinical signs. He was certainly brusque in his dealing with pa-

tients, but he was an expert in the field of diagnosis based on physical signs - in those days a much more important component of surgical practice than at the present time. In this area he taught postgraduates attending his clinic with enthusiasm, although it must be said with a certain degree of dogma. Looking back on those afternoons I spent in his clinic, I have no doubt that they were a considerable help to me in preparing for the Final FRCS.

The physician to whom Le Quesne refers was almost certainly Dr Punch, a small, neat and rather shortsighted man, whose medical clinic took place at the same time as Bailey's, in an adjoining room. Rex Lawrie was a House Surgeon at the Royal Northern during the Second World War and recalls that whenever a surgical opinion was required, and sometimes when it was not, Bailey would come into the room, tower over the patient and the diminutive physician, and offer to solve the problem by an operation. Dr Punch must have found these intrusions somewhat exasperating, but was in no position to complain.

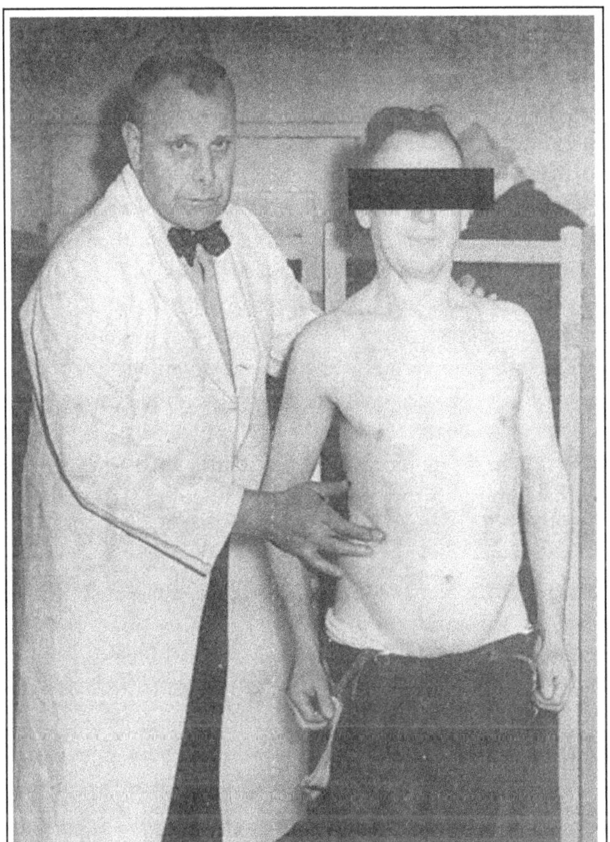

Figure 5.4: Bailey 'en brossse' demonstrates an examination of the abdomen of a patient

The Operating Theatre

The theatre staff came in early in the morning to make sure that the theatre was clean and that all the necessary instruments were laid out, under the supervision of the Theatre Sister who took tremendous pride in the running of her small domain (Bailey had his own set of insruments, many of which he had designed, and which no one else was allowed to use). The next to appear was the anaesthetist, who would check over his apparatus in readiness for the reception of the first patient. The surgeon's arrival was awaited with some trepidation. Bailey had a strict discipline in the operating theatre, and became angry if anything was not to his liking. For instance (as Rex Lawrie records) at certain stages in the operation he needed to have his brow wiped, and a trembling junior nurse would be summoned by Sister to do this for him. If she did not do it exactly right he would send her over into the corner of the theatre, there to practice wiping the forehead of some other nurse until she had mastered the technique - an ugly and embarassing experience not only for the young probationer but also for all others helping with the operation.

The most faithful anaesthetist was Dr Donald Blatchley. Quite soon after his arrival at the Royal Northern, Bailey had rescued Blatchley's wife from complications following a gynaecological operation, a debt which had never been forgotten, so that there was an affinity between the two men. Blatchley was known as a 'surgeon's anaesthetist' in that, if one of his colleagues had decided that an operation was necessary, he was always willing to help out, whatever his view of the case. In those days specialist anaesthetists were rare, so most anaesthetics were given by general practitioners or junior staff. Ian Robin was a houseman on another surgical firm at the Northern, but was quite often called upon to assist Bailey by giving an anaesthetic at some inconvenient time. John Elam was his anaesthetist at Potters Bar, and also occasionally at the Northern. Dr Elam was a strong and outspoken character, and there was immediate friction, until a mutual respect developed, as he discovered that Bailey 'had a heart of gold and did not know the meaning of the word jealousy. He did upset the nurses but when they got flustered I could always say "shut up, Ham" and he was all smiles'.

The lists generally consisted of two or three major cases (resection of the thyroid, stomach or gallbladder) followed by a number of intermediate or minor procedures such as repair of hernias, removal of small blemishes and opening of abscesses. There was an accent on urology, which had always been one of Bailey's major interests. First-hand accounts from those who worked with Bailey are unanimous that he was not a naturally gentle and dexterous surgeon. Figure 5.5 is the only surviving photograph of him in the operating theatre, and it is immediately obvious that there is a profusion of instruments around the operation field, and rather more bloodstained swabs than one would like to see. Good surgeons are neat, and this picture is a mess. He operated swiftly, and sometimes roughly. Ian Robin recollects that his entry into the abdomen was 'incredibly quick - inside in two minutes with the huge "London hooks" immediately inserted'. Humphreys records another of his house surgeons as saying: 'You will probably know something of his operating methods, very speedy, frequent accidents. On the whole he might have been better sticking to witing his books, which were excellent in every way. But we on the house felt that in a serious case Ham might well get away with success. He was often very fast. I remember a simple mastectomy that I was rushing to towel up, and he rushed even faster and with two big knife strokes he had the breast off before I could even start putting towels on'. Valentine Swain records his removing the breast and the uterus through

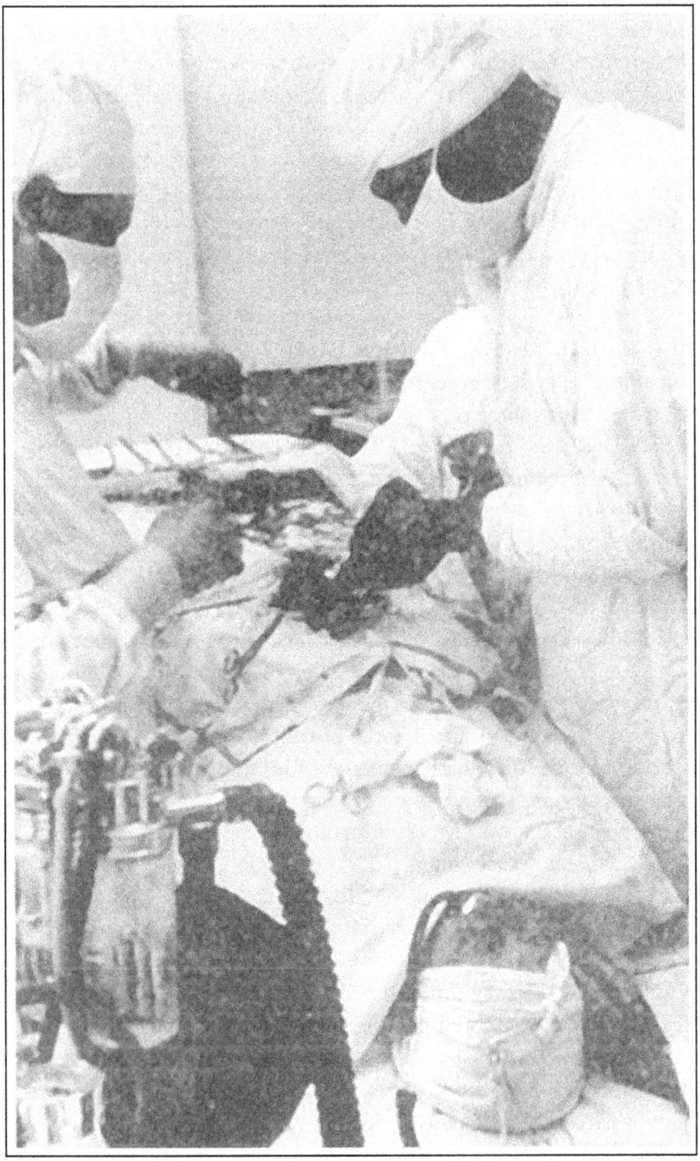

Figure 5.5: An operation at St Vincent's Clinic

one continuous incision running from the chest to the lower abdomen, the sort of colossal mutilation which attracted admiration at the time because of the overriding requirement to save the patient from prolonged anaesthesia.

Zina Fitzgerald was the daughter of the eminent paediatrician Alan Moncrieff who worked at the Hospital for Sick Children in Great Ormond Street and at The Middlesex, and was herself to become consultant paediatrician at the Royal Free Hospital. She was house surgeon at the Royal Northern in 1940 and spent a year there, in turn as house physician, house surgeon, out-patient medical officer and casualty officer. During her stay she met Freddy Fitzgerald, Bailey's orthopaedic colleague at the Northern, whom she later married. Although she never worked for Bailey she knew him well and used to give anaesthetics for his emergency cases. She remembers him as a man of unpredictable mood and a rapid and not always very accurate surgeon. One particular case comes to mind of an operation on the first rib which involved division of a blood vessel, from which the patient died from haemorrhage. (Presumably this was the subclavian artery.) He did not talk to his house officers and did not talk very much to his patients.

Alan Kark came to in 1944 and worked through 1945 and 1946 at the Royal Northern as house surgeon to W. G. Gabriel and to Hamilton Bailey. He remembers him as flamboyant, outgoing and friendly. He had private patients all over London and in Chatham and Potter's Bar, and Kark would help in this work. He was somewhat heavy handed as a surgeon and Kark remembers him rupturing an aortic aneurysm, which he had previously diagnosed as a tumour of the pancreas.

While all this gives the picture of a brutal and careless operator, it must be borne in mind that speed was a far more important consideration then than it is today, when smooth anaesthesia, muscle relaxing drugs and accurate monitoring of body functions have made operations so much easier and safer. The ether and chloroform available to the anaesthetist of the 1930s were powerful respiratory poisons, and the longer the patients were under their influence, the more difficult was their recovery. Bailey's speed enabled him to get through long operating lists, many times each week. More meticulous surgeons took a longer time over each case, and may have accomplished less work. He would undertake emergencies in very high risk patients, and would happily operate on advanced cancer. The word 'inoperable' was not part of his vocabulary.

Not only did he carry out two full days work at the Royal Northern, but also during this time he did regular sessions at Clacton on Sea, Oldchurch Hospital, Romford and Potters Bar, and occasional visits to Battersea, quite apart from emergencies and private practice. On alternate Saturday mornings, he was in the habit of travelling down to All Saints Hospital in Chatham where he would regularly carry out twelve operations.

The records of surgery at RNH extend from January 1931 to January 1947 (Figure 5.6). The first operation Bailey performed on his arrival was a removal of an ear for carcinoma on a Mrs Jane Truscott aged 81. This was exceptional, and although today surgery on the aged patient is commonplace, at that time the life expectancy was much briefer, and most surgical patients were two or three decades younger. The last operation he carried out was 2 January 1947 and consisted in opening the bladder under local anaesthestia for a 65 year-old-man with retention of urine. However, two days previously he is recorded as having operated upon a carotid body tumour. This is described a a 'first stage operation', so may have consisted of simply ligation of the external carotid artery. (N.B. On 26 September 1946 there is a note recording a total removal of the carotid bifurcation for a similar tumour, in a woman of 24. This operation would nowadays be considered highly dangerous and liable to lead to severe paralysis. The result is unknown.)

The work at Oldchurch extended from April 1932 to August 1939, that is nearly to the outbreak of the Second World War. Some 1500 operations were carried out during this time, again covering a wide variety of cases, but not including emergencies. Most of the problems were abdominal, with some orthopaedics and very little urology. Twelve cases of tuberculous lymphadenitis in the neck were treated, by Bailey's favoured method of wide excision and leaving the wound open to heal by granulation. There was surprisingly little surgery for peptic ulcer, with only a few gastrectomies or bypasses being recorded. Probably the commonest operation to be carried out in a present day National Health Service hospitals is for varicose veins, and it is remarkable that this everyday procedure is hardly ever mentioned in Bailey's operation books. Another extraordinary omission is that of parotidectomy. In spite of Bailey's reputed expertise in the surgery of the parotid gland, his authoritative writing and theories regarding the distribution of the facial nerve, the books which have survived mention only four of these operations, and there is no written record of his ever having performed a total removal of the gland. This is in spite of the fact that a typed note (presumably by Veta) on the front cover reads 'these two books contain a list of all the operations he ever performed'. However, Dr Elam who anaesthetised for him at Potters Bar records that he seemed to have one of these every week, and that he liked to do them as special cases on a Saturday morning. Perhaps that is why they seem to have escaped form the official record books.

Between March 1935 and October 1937 Bailey performed some 250 operations at Clacton on Sea. The theatre records show that he attended there once every two weeks, and the operations ranged from simple appendicectomies and hernia repairs, to radical mastectomy and intra-abdominal procedures for cancer. Each operation was carefully annotated according to the chapter of the book to which it was destined as for example the B (breast) GB (gallbladder) or T (thyroid). A certain number of orthopaedic procedures such as exploration of the hip and plating of fractures were also carried out. There were no emergencies.

During the Second World War (see below), Bailey had access to six EMS (Emergency Medical Service) beds at Potters Bar Hospital in Hertfordshire. He used to transfer patients from the Northern into these beds, to ease pressure on the main hospital, which was receiving air raid casualties (and later casualties from flying bombs) at some 50 per month. However when the authorities at Potters Bar became aware of this practice they raised objections and insisted that

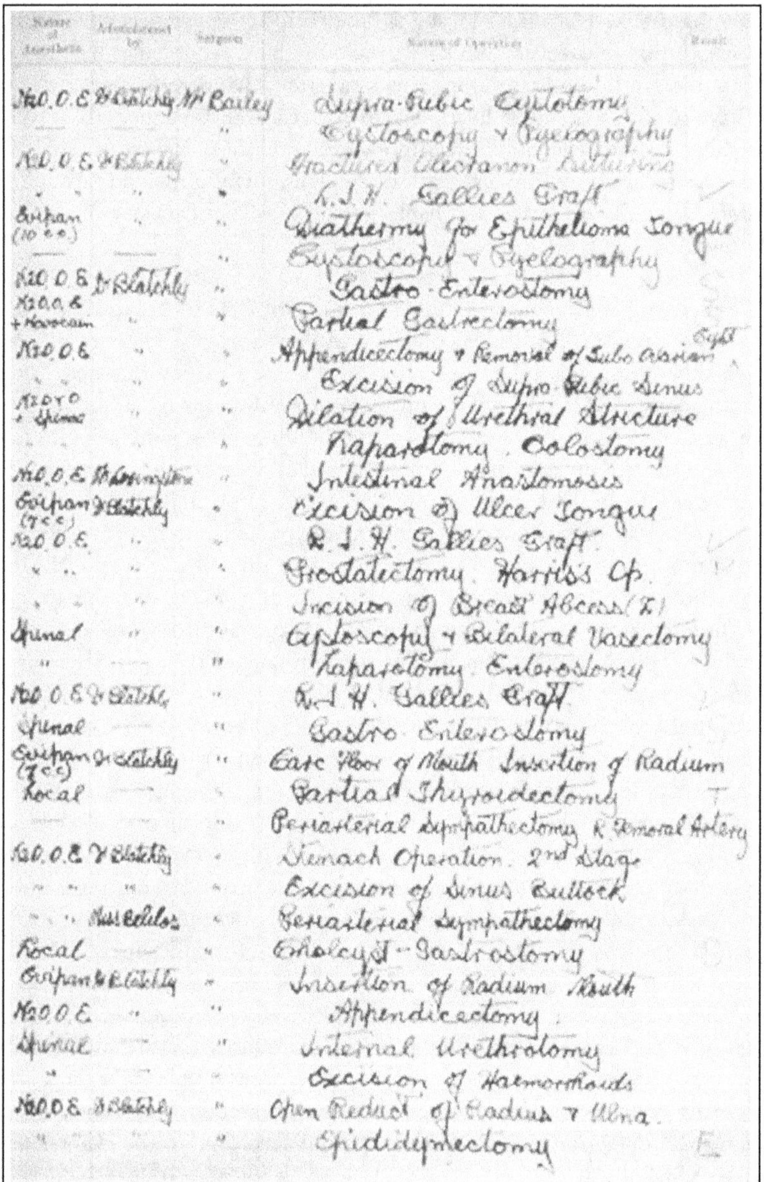

Nature of Anaesthetic	Administered by	Surgeon	Nature of Operation	Result
N2O. O. E.	Dr Blatchly	Mr Bailey	Supra-Pubic Cystotomy	
		"	Cystoscopy & Pyelography	
N2O. O. E.	Dr Blatchly	"	Fractured Olecranon Suturing	
"	"	"	R. J. H. Gallies Graft	
Evipan (10 c.c.)	"	"	Diathermy for Epithelioma Tongue	
		"	Cystoscopy & Pyelography	
N2O. O. E.	Dr Blatchly	"	Gastro-Enterostomy	
N2O. O. E. + Novocain	"	"	Partial Gastrectomy	
N2O. O. E.	"	"	Appendicectomy & Removal of Sub-Ovarian Cyst	
"	"	"	Excision of Supra-Pubic Sinus	
N2O & O + Spinal	"	"	Dilation of Urethral Stricture	
"	"	"	Laparotomy. Colostomy	
N2O. O. E.	Dr [illegible]	"	Intestinal Anastomosis	
Evipan (7 c.c.)	Dr Blatchly	"	Excision of Ulcer Tongue	
N2O. O. E.	"	"	R. J. H. Gallies Graft	
"	"	"	Prostatectomy. Harris's Op.	
"	"	"	Incision of Breast Abscess (L)	
Spinal	"	"	Cystoscopy & Bilateral Vasectomy	
"		"	Laparotomy. Enterostomy	
N2O. O. E.	Dr Blatchly	"	R. J. H. Gallies Graft	
Spinal		"	Gastro-Enterostomy	
Evipan (7 c.c.)	Dr Blatchly	"	Ca. Floor of Mouth Insertion of Radium	
Local		"	Partial Thyroidectomy	
		"	Periarterial Sympathectomy R Femoral Artery	
N2O. O. E.	Dr Blatchly	"	Stomach Operation. 2nd Stage	
"	"	"	Excision of Sinus Buttock	
"	Miss [illegible]	"	Periarterial Sympathectomy	
Local		"	Cholecyst-Gastrostomy	
Evipan	Dr Blatchly	"	Insertion of Radium Mouth	
N2O. O. E.	"	"	Appendicectomy	
Spinal		"	Internal Urethrotomy	
"		"	Excision of Haemorrhoids	
N2O. O. E.	Dr Blatchly	"	Open Reduct. of Radius & Ulna	
"		"	Epididymectomy	

Figure 5.6: The Theatre record from the Royal Northern Hospital

services (he used to visit the hospital every two weeks) were used for the benefit of local patients. In all, Bailey performed 1122 operations at Potters Bar between September 1941 and January 1947. Humphreys spoke to a nurse who had known him there and who declared: 'He worked 18 hours out of a 24-hour day, but he was the most unpopular surgeon we ever had...he was a genius himself and had no time for anyone who was slow...'

He also was appointed to the Italian Hospital, although there is nothing to suggest that he spoke a word of that language. The hospital closed in 1941 when Italy entered the war, but re-opened in 1946 and continued working for the next years. In the interim, much of the work was transferred to the St Vincent's Clinic. The elegant dome of the Ospedale Italiano in Queen Square still stands, and although its trustees still operate for the benefit of the Italian comunity in London, the clinical and business records have been destroyed.

It is possible to tell from these operation books how many operations were performed on each day of the week, though not (as was the case at Dudley Road) at what time of day. For example, page 80 shows that on the 1 January 1943 he carried a hernia repair, an appendicectomy, a skin graft and a retrograde pyelogram, and the following week there was a excision of tuberculous glands of the neck, a partial thyroidectomy and an appendicectomy. As well as this work outside his main hospital he was completing two full-day operating lists each week at the Royal Northern. It seems that virtually all of these operations were charitable, his remunerative private practice being carried out at St Vincent's Clinic and, later, at the Lambeth Nursing Home.

What is harder to assess is the result of these operations, as such outcome records as were taken have been lost. Occasionally there is a cryptic entry (usually in pencil and in another handwriting) which says 'died', giving a time and date shortly after the operation. Many of the procedures are described as 'radical cure' which looks impressive but is an over optimistic description of outcome. This phrase is most particularly applied to the treatment of inguinal hernia, and we know that the recurrence rate of hernia repair in the first half of the century approached 15%. There are two pieces of evidence which mitigate Bailey's reputation as a poor technician. In the first place, the results of treatment, and particularly bad results, are quickly known, and if the outcome of his surgery had been consistently unsatisfactory he would never have achieved the scale of referrals from the local general practitioners which in fact he did. Secondly, the 'reoperation' rate of a particular surgeon is very revealing in this regard. If the same patient's name crops up in the theatre record several times during one week, for example a radical operation on a Tuesday, returned to theatre for bleeding on Wednesday, Friday resuturing of wound, etc., this gives an insight into the level of technical ability. The 'returned to theatre' rate in Bailey's operative record is very low. However, this figure must be interpreted with some caution. Because he was always on the move, it could not have been easy to make contact with Bailey and summon him back to the operating theatre if something had gone wrong, and the Registrar (or even perhaps a houseman or GP) would be expected to clear up the mess. Again, because of the lack of blood for transfusion, and the ignorance of the principles of resuscitation, the concept of 'post operative shock' was accepted as an inevitable consequence of surgery rather than an indication for prompt remedial action, and many patients who nowadays would be taken back to the theatre to have a complication put right, were at that time given up for lost. The operating books only record the operations which Bailey carried out, and a subsequent attempt by a Registrar or HS to stop bleeding or repair a suture line would not appear.

Many of the procedures reflect the surgical practice of the 1930s and would not be performed today. These include operations for correction of such supposed abnormalities as dropped stomach or kidneys ('gastropexy' and 'nephropexy'), the Gallie fascial graph for hernia repair, and peri-arterial sympathectomy for arterial disease. There are many recordings of operations for chronic appendicitis, a disease which was fashionable at the time, but probably has no basis in pathology. The 'grumbling appendix' was a convenient diagnostic label to explain away recurrent abdominal pains in (particularly) young women and, a cynic might say, this simple operation to remove a normal organ provided a useful and trouble-free means of adding to a surgeon's income. But Bailey commanded loyalty. A doctor from New Zealand lost a finger in almost identical circumstances to Bailey, through removing a septic appendix, and many years later, having read an account of Bailey's problem, asked for his help because of a painful nerve. There result was a comfortable, slim hand.

All in all, whatever the value of his overall contribution to surgical science, the verdict on Bailey's technical ability must be unfavourable. Two questions suggest themselves. Firstly, if he was in truth a poor operator, how did he achieve his career and hold down responsible posts? And again, if his results were unsatisfactory, how was he allowed to remain there? It is often assumed that surgeons undergo some form of manual assessment test, and are selected on grounds of dexterity, but this is not so. Diagnostic ability, decisiveness, the capacity to know when not to operate, communication skills and organisational talents, are all in themselves important parts of training, of the selection process and in the exercise of the profession, and Bailey had all of these. Again, it was very difficult to removed a consultant once appointed, and to an extent that is still the case. The same, of course, applies to judges, managing directors and others. If Bailey's surgery had been scandalously below standard, he would have been exposed in the Courts, but this never happened. Deaths within 24 hours of operation, then as now, are required by law to be reported to the Coroner, and Ian Robin remembers attending the Coroner's Court quite frequently following the death of one of Bailey's patients. In the climate of the 1930s the surgeon was seldom blamed, but rather applauded for the efforts he had made to save life against difficult odds, but Coroners then as now were watchful of repeated mistakes. The fact is that Bailey was probably no worse a technician than many surgeons of his generation, and certainly worked a good deal harder than most of them. If one was asked the question, 'as a patient in North London in the 1930s, would you have chosen Bailey for your surgeon?' the answer would probably be no. But it would be wrong to deny the contribution which he made, however indirectly, to many generations of sick people.

The End of the Day

At the end of the day he would return to Fairlawn where Veta would have arranged some hospitality for the local medical profession or for foreign visitors. She would not allow him to join the gathering until he had at first completed his notes, changed into a respectable suit of clothes, and signed the letters and records, retrieved from the morning's wax cylinder. Quite often, another cylinder would have been filled up, resulting from his activities during the second half of the day, and this would be left for the secretaries to deal with later. Bailey would try to join the festivities, from loyalty to Veta and also because he recognised that this was an essential part of his practice, but quite often he became so bored with the social scene that after a perfunctory greeting to his colleagues and visitors he would go back to his study and continue work on books and papers. Although there was plenty of food and drink around at Fairlawn, Bailey was very abstemious, except in the matter of tobacco. He took an occasional small whisky, but unlike many of his colleagues he had absolutely no dependence on alcohol. He did however smoke very heavily, and used to break off between operations for a cigarette.

Back in the study, he would meet his favourite pets, not the dogs or cats who shared the house, but a collection of tropical fish in a heated tank. He liked them because they were colourful but at the same time made no noise. But he was not free from disturbance. Night-time emergency calls were quite frequent, and were usually dealt with in person, even if that required a journey out to some distant hospital. Veta's dinner parties tended to be disturbed by the sound of a heavy Rolls Royce crunching off down the driveway. Next morning, the working day would begin again, with the cold plunge. No concession was made to weekends: Saturday mornings were devoted to operating lists in Chatham or elsewhere, and Sundays to writing. Both the Baileys played a little golf, and belonged to a local club, but attendance was somewhat half-hearted, and one has the impression that membership was really a matter of conformity and an opportunity to make contact with potentially useful colleagues.

Chapter 6

THE SECOND WORLD WAR AND INTERNATIONAL FAME

Islington at War

There had always been undergraduate students at the Northern, and volunteers from St Bartholomew's and The Middlesex helped to place sandbags around the hospital in the few days before the first Sunday in September 1939, when the Second World War broke out. An underground operating theatre was organised including two tables, sterilising and anaesthetic rooms, the surgeons' room and the store room. Independent lighting was provided by a traction engine and dynamo brought down from Hampstead Heath. At the request of the Ministry of Health, 150 beds were made available in Wards 4, 5 and 6, and Dr Green's radiotherapy department was converted to receive casualties. Sixty nurses and sisters from the Royal Northern were sent out to Barnet to help staff the hospitals there, although many of them subsequently came back, and almost all of the consultants from the Northern, including Bailey, worked in both hospitals and took it in turns to sleep in. Additionally, a mobile surgical team was organised consisting of a consultant and an assistant consultant surgeon, anaesthetist, theatre sister and theatre attendant. A first-aid post was set up in the Outpatient department and the fracture clinic was converted into a gas cleansing station.

In point of fact, none of these carefully prepared facilities was ever called into use. This was the period of the 'Phoney War' which lasted up until the fall of France and the beginning of the Battle of Britain. At the end of 1940, the Ministry of Health reassessed the situation and released many of the beds which had been reserved for casualties, back to general civilian use. St David's Wing and the main floors were reopened, and private patients as well as civilian and service emergency cases and some air raid casualties were admitted and cared for by the surgical teams, among whom Bailey was particularly active. The hospital was fortunate enough to escape a direct hit, although at one point it was deprived of mains electricity and water because of damage to underground drains and cables. On the night of 26 September 1940, a bomb fell behind the circular wards and demolished the boiler house and linen store, but there were no casualties, and the damage was quickly repaired. Other hospitals were not so lucky. The Royal Chest Hospital was destroyed, and many of their patients and staff were transferred to the Northern, which as a result received much help from the King Edward's Fund, the British Red Cross, and most particularly from the American Red Cross Committee, who sent generous donations of money, instruments and clothing through the 'Bundles for Britain' scheme. The Chairman of the Governors, Lord Bessborough, acknowledging a gift of $10,000, sent a telegram to The Chairman of the American Society on 16 January 1941, which read:

> *I send this profound message of gratitude to all donors in America from the management, doctors and nurses at The Royal Northern Hospital, for friendship, sympathy and practical assistance to our damaged hospital. This spontaneous and generous gift will help to save many lives and increase aid to the sick and injured in our bombed city.*

Back in Totteridge, with domestic and secretarial staff being called up, and no one to tend a large garden, Fairlawn became impossible to manage and in 1941 the Baileys moved to a smaller house a mile down the road, called 'Denham'. It was not a particularly safe area, and Veta and Hamilton are on record as crouching together in the basement of their new home, busily compiling the latest book, while bombs fell around them.

The Books

Rex Lawrie recounts the following anecdote. Over a cup of coffee, a visitor to the RNH operating theatre asked Bailey how he wrote his books. 'It is perfectly straightforward', was the reply, 'you think of a number of chapter titles, send them round to a number of celebrated names, and when they send in their contributions you illustrate them lavishly and rewrite them'. 'Don't they mind?' asked the visitor. 'Well, no. By the time the book is printed they have forgotten what they wrote anyway. There was one little whippersnapper in Norwich who wrote and complained'. (Lawrie identifies the whippersnapper as a respected orthopaedic surgeon named H. A. Brittain).

While this cynical policy might have been applied to the later books, it was certainly not a possibility when Bailey started as an unknown registrar in Birmingham. *Physical Signs in Clinical Surgery*, Bailey's first book, which had appeared in 1927, had run to six editions by the outbreak of the war. *Emergency Surgery* was in its fifth edition and *Short Practice*, written with McNeill Love, in its fourth. Work on the books continued during the war. Many of Bailey's young assistants and disciples were now away in the Western Desert, in Greece and Crete and Burma, encountering at first hand the sort of experience of traumatic surgery which Bailey had not met since the Battle of Jutland. Reports from his juniors all over the world flooded in to the house in Totteridge, sometimes together with photographs, which were carefully studied and touched up by Veta. The senior editor of the medical publishers E. & S. Livingstone of Edinburgh, Charles MacMillan, realised early in the war that an authoritative text book on the management of battle injuries would be urgently required, and felt that the only man able to produce this at short notice was Bailey. He wrote:

> *I simply longed to meet and get to know this amazing medical author. I used to watch him when his car was held up in London's busy traffic. He worked hard between appointments, either private or at various hospitals, widely scattered, where he was on the staff. Oblivious to what was happening in the busy streets or country lanes, he could be seen working on his Dictaphone which was suitably installed in his spacious Rolls Royce. Everyday he must write something. He always sets himself a target, usually obtained by sheer determination and discipline. Both Mr Hamilton Bailey and his wife were enthusiastic about our proposition. In a few months a team of contributors was arranged, then the first part of one hundred and twenty eight pages was on sale. Hard work was involved but it was a magnificent publishing achievement. During the war years on many occasions the City was frequently bombed I stayed at his lovely home in Totteridge. In discussions I learnt the secret of his success as a medical author. A presentation must be perfect and lavishly illustrated.*

The product of this experience was *The Surgery of Modern Warfare*, published in Edinburgh in 1940, a remarkable achievement bearing in mind that the book was written by a man who was far from the battlefield, and was working day and night under great difficulties. It was quickly adopted as an authoritative text, and was issued to directors of medical services at divisional and regimental levels (DDMS & ADMS). For many years after the end of the war, it remained the official surgical textbook for the Royal Army Medical Corps. Of all its messages, perhaps the one which has saved most lives is the chapter on delayed primary suture (DPS).

The concept of DPS is very simple. An injury sustained by a soldier on the battlefield is far more serious and life threatening than a clean wound created by a surgeon, or accidentally by a sharp knife in the kitchen, because it almost always contains contaminated foreign bodies such as bullet fragments or clothing, together with dead or threatened tissue, which inevitably leads to bacterial infection resulting in suppuration, gangrene and often loss of a limb or a life. Confronted by a gaping wound, common sense suggests that it should forthwith be sewn up, but on a battlefield this is disastrous, because it imprisons a mass of poisonous material in the injured body. The correct management of a war wound is to clean it thoroughly and to remove all the dead and damaged tissue and foreign material (which may involve a very radical operation) and then to leave it wide open, providing a clean surface upon which the normal defence mechanisms of the body can get to work, helped of course by appropriate antibiotics. A few days later, the whole area is usually found to healthy, and can be safely repaired. Obviously, if contamination remains, the cleansing process has to be repeated.

This simple concept, developed in 1914-18 and rediscovered in the Spanish Civil War, so clear and so obvious, and so beneficial in its outcome, as stressed by Bailey and others, has been repeatedly ignored. During the Second World War and the Korean and Vietnam campaigns, and later in Somalia and Rwanda, many battlefield wounds were closed on the spot, with disastrous consequences. These mistakes have been projected into civilian life. Young doctors in accident and emergency departments, and young surgeons in training, ignorant of these painfully learned principles, will occasionally introduce tight stitches into wounds incurred on building sites or in road traffic accidents. The results are as bad as ever.

By now, *A Short Practice of Surgery* has sold more than 400,000 copies in the English language alone, and has achieved by far the largest circulation of any book on surgery ever written. The first three editions were well received, but the fourth, for some reason, attracted a very hostile review from the *Guy's Hospital Gazette*. 'The student would be well advised to avoid this book', thundered the critic. 'Like the devil incarnate, its outward appearance is good, but it must inevitably lead to disaster'. The review was widely quoted and may well have stimulated sales. Although of course much altered, *Short Practice* is now in its 21st edition, and is still known all over the world as 'Bailey and Love', though contemporary witnesses say that the writing was 90% Bailey and 10% Love. Years later, Allan Clain discovered that whereas Bailey (or perhaps Veta) was always ready to update a chapter, it was difficult to hold McNeill Love to any deadline. In point of fact, Love had some years before written a book called *A Shorter Surgery*, which to his great disappointment had been turned down by the publishers, so that Bailey had little difficulty in persuading him to incorporate it in the new work.

McNeill Love

Although they known each other ever since their registrar days at the London in the 1920s, and Love had taken the trouble to visit and encourage his colleague during the bleak time in Birmingham, the two never became close friends, and on the rare occasions when they met they addressed each other by their surnames. Robert McNeill Love was three years older than Bailey, and had been born of old Northern Irish stock. His father, a successful warehouseman, had bought the former home of Scott of the Antarctic on the Antrim coast, where he raised his close-knit and affectionate family. Love qualified in 1914 and immediately joined the army, serving throughout the war in Turkey and the Middle East. Apart from his war service, he never moved out of London and before joining the staff at the Royal Northern his only appontments had been at the Metropolitan and the Mildmay Mission Hospitals in the East End. With this sedate background Love was a very different character from his colleague, not only being a more sympathetic man, but also by all accounts being a calmer and technically neater surgeon. A devout Anglican, upright, self effacing and dutiful, spending his week ends as a Commissioner for Scouts and Guides (for whom he had bought a playing field out of his savings), Love commanded the sort of affection from his patients, nurses and medical colleagues which Bailey never achieved. He was not entirely free from vanity, as he continued to dye his greying hair, a fact which was noted with quiet amusement by his friends but never alluded to in his presence. Having been Chairman of the Court of Examiners of the Royal College of Surgeons for a number of years he was elected a member of the Council in 1945, and on his retirement in 1953 endowed the McNeill Love medal, which is awarded to a member of the staff of the College who has served for 25 years in a capacity other than that of a senior academic or administrator. It was typical of him that he sought to acknowledge the services of the inconspicuous. Love's first wife died when she was quite young. He then lost a son through renal tuberculosis, though whether he and Bailey ever saw this as a point of shared sympathy remains doubtful. In later life, becoming lonely, Love advertised for a housekeeper in a magazine called *The Lady*, adding that 'if all goes well, marriage might follow'. The advertisement was answered by Rhoda, the widow of a Bristol clergyman, and indeed all did go well. The pair lived happily for many years, until Love died on 1 October 1974 from cancer of the stomach, 80 years to the day following Bailey's birth. His Medal continues to be awarded by the College which he served so well.

One of the unique features of the Bailey textbooks is the faithful acknowledgement of names and sources. Thus, throughout *Short Practice*, whenever an operation or discovery is mentioned, there is a footnote stating who was responsible, and giving his or her (there were no women surgeons in the early days) dates of birth and death, position and country of origin - a convention that has persisted right up to the 21st edition, which appeared in 1994. Some of these footnotes are engagingly trivial. For instance, in the discussion of broken jaws in the first edition there is a reference to the Gunning Splint, and at the bottom of the page we discover that Thomas Brian Gunning (1811-89) was

> *... a dentist from 'New York, USA', the inventor of a remarkably fashioned vulcanite plate which was used to set the fractured mandible of William H. Seward, President Abraham Lincoln's Secretary of State.*

How Bailey came upon this sensationally unimportant piece of information we shall never know, but those of us who delight in small things are grateful to him and to succeeding Editors who have faithfully recorded them over the years, and hope that they will take care not to omit such gems in future volumes.

From these footnotes, and with the help of W. J. Bishop, the librarian of the Royal Society of Medicine, Bailey was able to compile a small book - *Notable Names in Medicine and Surgery* (Figure 6.1) which is a collection of potted biographies and vignettes, with plenty of pictures, beginning with Hippocrates and finishing up with the then Professor of Surgery at Toronto. Carl Krebs, in an obituary, records his satisfaction at the inclusion of four distinguished Danes. *Notable Names* first appeared in 1944 and ran into six editions. It is a delightful little book, unusually light hearted for Bailey, and still a useful reference.

There were two editions of *101 Demonstrations of Surgery for Nurses* which appeared during the war years.

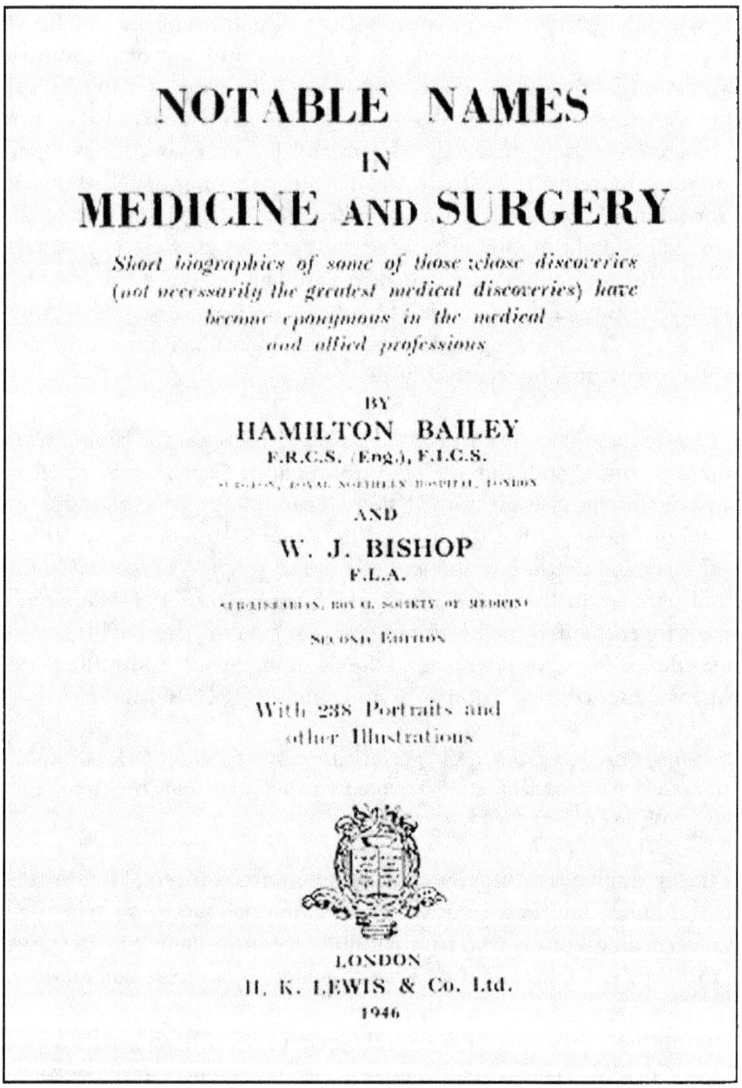

NOTABLE NAMES
IN
MEDICINE AND SURGERY

Short biographies of some of those whose discoveries (not necessarily the greatest medical discoveries) have become eponymous in the medical and allied professions

BY
HAMILTON BAILEY
F.R.C.S. (Eng.), F.I.C.S.

AND
W. J. BISHOP
F.L.A.

SECOND EDITION

With 238 Portraits and other Illustrations

LONDON
H. K. LEWIS & Co. Ltd.
1946

Figure 6.1: Notable Names, *2nd edn (1946)*

International Activity

Short Practice, *Physical Signs* and *Emergency Surgery* had all been translated into various European languages. Contact with European colleagues, in particular with his old friend Carl Krebs from Denmark, continued up to the beginning of the war. Of all the societies to which Bailey belonged, the only one which he really enjoyed was the American-founded International College of Surgeons. This is easy to understand as he spoke no other language than English, so was unable to contribute to a French or German meeting, but at the same time did not feel at ease or accepted by his colleagues in England. He abhorred formal dinners and ceremonial occasions, felt uneasy in committees, and his experiences in Liverpool and Birmingham had made him wary of medical politics. Although in 1949 he was awarded a Hunterian Professorship of the Royal College of Surgeons (giving a discourse on parotidectomy), he never stood for election to the Council, and did not even gain a place on its Court of Examiners, the body responsible for awarding the FRCS diploma. (Scotland, however, recognised Bailey's achievement, by electing him a Fellow of the Royal Society of Edinburgh in 1946.) In contrast with the standoffish attitudes of his compatriots, the relaxed and democratic nature of the American surgical fraternity was a natural refuge, where he felt understood and appreciated.

The International College of Surgeons had been the idea of Max Thorek. Thorek was born in Hungary in 1880 and emigrated to the USA as a penniless refugee in 1900. He enrolled as a student at Rush Medical College in Chicago, and graduated MD in 1904. He wrote extensively, drawing on his experience as attending surgeon to the Cook County Hospital, one of the largest public Hospitals in the USA, which dealt with a vast range of surgical illnesses. Thorek was enthusiastic about international co-operation between surgeons, wishing to combine the accumulated historical wisdom and experience of Europe with the dynamism and technical skills of his adopted country. He was instrumental in creating the International College in 1935, appointing himself as Secretary General and Treasurer, but leaving the Presidency to Arnold Jirasek from Prague. The first Executive Secretary/Treasurer from Europe was Hamilton Bailey who continued under the next President, Dr Crotti from Cincinnati. Bailey's books were by now known world-wide, and he must have been pleased that the lack of recognition in his own country was now compensated in the rest of the world. The College published a journal, at first called the *Transactions of the ICS* (to which Bailey contributed an article on the transverse upper abdominal incision) later the *Journal of International Surgery*, and finally simply *International Surgery*. Bailey was Assistant Editor of all three, and wrote in all 20 contributions for them.

As the Second World War continued, professional contacts between American and European surgeons became more difficult, not only due to the dangers of transatlantic sea travel, but also because the needs of the battlefield pushed basic research into such problems as cancer and deformity into second place, at least as far as the Europeans were concerned. There was also a dilemma as to the stance which American surgeons, many of whom had German or Italian forebears, should take up vis-à-vis the European conflict. As rumours about the fate of European Jewry began to emerge, attitudes hardened, and at the Conference in 1943 following America's entry into the war, at which Bailey spoke on crush syndrome and McNeill Love on gas gangrene, it was agreed not to translate the proceedings into German or Italian. A number of Russian colleagues were welcomed, though no one was able to understand, still less translate, their papers. In retrospect, it seems strange that Bailey and Love should have been allowed to leave Britain in the middle of the war, to attend such a meeting, particularly since both were badly needed at home The Medical Committee minutes of the time do not record their absence, and perhaps there were security reasons for that omission.

After the war, the ICS held meetings in Chicago (1947), Rome (1948) and in New York in 1950, which coincided with Max Thorek's 70th birthday. On that occasion McNeill Love wrote "Twelve years after reading Max Thorek's article on the technique of cholecystectomy, my colleague Hamilton Bailey and I adopted the technique he devised, and have reported 129 cases without mortality."

Curiously, in spite of Bailey's initiative, it was not until 1962, a year after his death, that the British section of the International College of Surgeons was founded. Although the ICS still exists, it can no longer claim to have much influence on surgical practice. It originated as an organisation of general surgeons, but science and society have moved on. In the developed world, general surgeons are a vanishing species. People now expect to be treated by a specialist in their particular disorder, and often have read intensively and know a great deal about it. Whereas in Bailey's day to be a general surgeon was the acme of success, and to specialise in otolaryngology or orthopaedics was seen as accepting a second level post where the competition was less intense, nowadays the general surgeon is coming to be seen somewhat as a Jack of all Trades, much as Lord Moran viewed the lowly GP of the early years of this century. This is certainly the trend in Western Europe and North America, with the result that organisations such as the ICS tend to rely for support on countries whose medicine is less well-developed.

Young Hamilton

Men of Bailey's generation had in their younger years been accustomed to the realities of war, and reacted coolly to bombs or threats of invasion. Many of them signed up to join the Home Guard ('Dad's Army') or volunteered as Air Raid Wardens, directing people to shelters, clearing débris and putting out fires on London's rooftops. Doctors such as Bailey who were too old to fight were recruited into the Emergency Medical Service. Many of them had sons serving abroad, and bereavement was a shared fact of life. But what happened to Hamilton and Veta Bailey in 1943 was an experience which was so uniquely grotesque as to be unsharable.

Young Hamilton had always been thoughtful and well-behaved, and when he was a small baby seldom woke his mother from sleep. His upbringing had been rather restless, as his parents moved from place to place, and Veta had employed nursemaids to look after him when she was preoccupied with her husband's books. This was typical of her sense of priorities. As soon as he was of school age, he was dispatched to a prep school in Kent, no doubt rather similar to 'Durley'.

When the family moved to London, he was entered for Mill Hill School, where he spent two very happy years. At home, young Hamilton (Figure 6.2) was a rather shy and reclusive boy, who had difficulty in relating to his father, which perhaps reflects Bailey's earlier experience in Brighton.

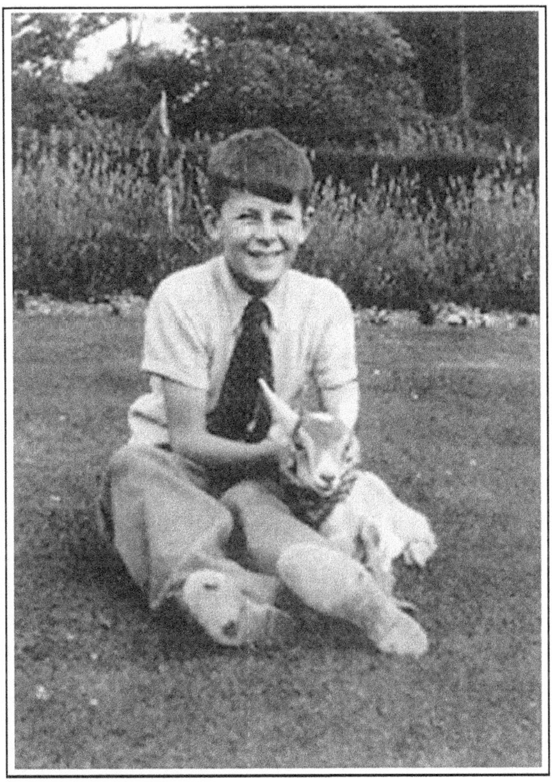

Figure 6.2: Young Hamilton with his pet goat

Whether by choice or by parental order, he rarely attended the social evenings at Fairlawn, but was expected to get up and share the icy plunge into the swimming pool. A wartime guest recorded:

> *Young Hamilton joined us at the water's edge. I asked him if he liked it. 'No, I hate it. But if you knew the Guv'nor you'd understand'.*

Even as long ago as 1940, it was weirdly exceptional for a boy to refer to his father as 'the Guv'nor'. Although they shared their first name (again, something unusual even in those days) young Hamilton physically resembled his mother, with whom he felt close and at ease.

In contrast to his home personality, at school Hamilton was a popular extrovert, a fine cricketer and renowned as a raconteur. He shared his father's disregard for money, and if his mother forgot to supply him with pocket money he in turn would forget to ask for it. A contemporary relates that 'he used to give us all nightmares in the dormitory since he was a good storyteller and told widely exaggerated and macabre tales about the emergency operations that his father had carried out using their carving knife on the kitchen table. The stories of what his father did with the bits that were left over at the end of the operations are not repeatable here but showed an inventive turn of mind'. Young Hamilton's parents were too busy to entertain children, so that not many of his friends from the dormitory saw him at home.

At the outbreak of the war, London schools were evacuated from the capital, so as to remove the children from the anticipated German bombardment. Mill Hill was allocated to the seaside town of St Bees in Cumbria. The school records show that the transfer was moderately successful and that most of the London boys settled happily into their new surroundings. They were accommodated in various boarding houses around the town. Hamilton was given a 'study' in Seacroft House, which was one of those used by Mill Hill school. The room was in fact a converted loose box in a stable, which he shared with two others. The horses were probably evacuated to better accommodation.

Although during term time they were protected from the London Blitzkrieg, the boys nonetheless returned to their homes for the holiday period, and on 29 July 1943 at the end of the Spring term, young Hamilton and his friends boarded the school special form Carlisle to London, under the charge of their housemaster, Mr J. P. Morrison, for the Easter break, bombs or no bombs. The train was full of happy schoolboys, who accepted the nightly blackout, the searchlights over their skies, the air raid sirens and their parents' preoccupation with battlefield casualties, as a part of normal life. Indeed, most of them had known nothing else since reaching the age of awareness. In spite of Hitler's recent successes, morale in the country was high.

The train service from Cumbria to London was owned and managed by the London Midland and Scottish (LMS) railway. There were two classes of travel, which were called first and third. There had originally been three classes, but the second class had proved uneconomical and had been eliminated many years before. Most countries would have chosen to rename the lower class accommodation as 'second', which would have a clear promotional advantage, but the British, as usual, clung to their history and arrived at an individual solution, in line with driving on the left side of the road, a twelve figure currency, and measurements in ounces, pints and furlongs, so that first and third class travel it remained.

Schoolboys always travelled third class, and in fact there was not much difference between the two sorts of carriage except as regards lighting and footroom. Corridor trains were virtually unknown, except on the Pullman service operating in continental Europe, so that the compartments were quite separate. Each contained two rows of four seats, facing each other, and a central door, opening outwards on to the track, and operated by an iron handle for the lock, and a heavy perforated leather strap for the window. The window and the door functioned quite separately. Thus it was possible to manipulate the metal handle of the door and swing it outwards, or else to keep the door closed and haul upwards on the leather strap, and then lean out of the window. There was a notice just below the ledge which read 'It is Dangerous to Lean out of the Window'. Young Hamilton's friends either did not read such notices, or if they did, saw them as a challenge. One can picture the scene of a carriage full of recently liberated adolescent boys, coming home to London for their holidays, fighting each other in the compartment, and opening the doors and windows in order to throw out toffee papers and apple cores and shout insults at the passers by. This end of term ritual was stoically accepted by the railway staff as a thrice yearly annoyance. In fact, on this particular occasion, Mr Morrison recorded that the boys were unusually quiet and well-behaved, although the Guard had had occasion to warn them not to lean out of the window. Just north of Preston, the train drew to a halt, and young Hamilton who was with three other boys in the fifth compartment of the third coach from the front of the train, leaned out to see what was happening. In the compartment immediately ahead was his friend Peter Bennett, of Torquay, who was also leaning out. A northbound goods train came slowly alongside, and Peter noticed that two of its doors were partly open. He tried to grab the handle of the first door in order to shut it but missed his hold, and as the door came up to Hamilton's window he tried to do the same, missed, and the door swung wide open and struck him a colossal mutilating blow to the head.

Hamilton fell back into the carriage, into the midst of his appalled young friends, pouring blood from a shattered neck, and virtually decapitated. There was no telephone, and apart from the communication cord ('Penalty £5 for Improper Use') no means of summoning anyone in authority. For whatever reason, the shaken boys did not pull the cord, and the train travelled on into Preston Station, where they tumbled out on to the platform and blurted out the dreadful news to the schoolmasters and the platform staff. The carriage was disconnected, and young Hamilton's body was taken out and placed in a nearby mortuary. After brief formalities, the rest of the train continued on its way. One can barely imagine the atmosphere in the coach reserved for Mill Hill boys, and the desperate efforts of the accompanying teachers to restore some atmosphere of calm. The train arrived at Euston many hours late, where the waiting parents had been told that an accident had occurred, but did not know of its nature. Instead of the noisy crowd of young schoolboys leaping out to begin their summer holidays, they encountered a quiet, pale group, many of whom were in tears.

In the meantime, Hamilton's identity being quickly confirmed, the police contacted Veta at Denham. We do not know how the message was delivered, still less how it was received. It might even have been communicated by a telegram, delivered at her house by a messenger boy on a printed slip with words such as 'Your son unfortunately dead in train accident. Condolences. Preston Police' (Figure 6.3).

In any event, we do know that Hamilton Bailey was operating at Potters Bar at the time, and that Veta was alone in the house when the message arrived. She telephoned the hospital secretary insisting that the news should be delivered by somebody in a senior position, who knew Bailey well, and could choose the time and mode of breaking it to him. This went disastrously wrong. The message was given to a junior employee outside the operating theatre, who struggled into sterile clothing, rushed up to the table and blurted out an account of his son's death to Bailey, who having completed a delicate operation for undescended testes, was in the midst of a gallbladder dissection. Swain records that he received the news with icy calm, completed the operation and called for the next case.

"SCHOOLBOYS' EXPRESS" FATALITY AT PRESTON

A Mill Hill (London) schoolboy. Hamilton Bailey (15), evacuated from London to St. Bees College, Cumberland, was killed on the L.M.S. at Preston to-day.

It is understood that he was leaning out of a carriage window of a "schoolboys" special when he was struck by a passing train.

Henry Airey (29), general dealer, of Leeds, was fined £2 15s. expenses for ill-treating a horse by working it in an unfit sate, at Leck.

Figure 6.3: From the Lancashire Daily Post, *29 July 1943*

Insensitive, uncaring, arrogant? There was no one there for him to hand over to, and professional ethic dictated that whatever the surgeon's personal circumstances, the interests of the patient, helpless on the operating table, must have priority. Moreover, for someone of Bailey's temperament to have abandoned what he was doing, give vent to his emotions and find the words to comfort his wife, was too difficult to contemplate. He was simply not ready for it. It was easier to continue with something that, although requiring concentration, was familiar, and provided him with time to absorb the news and to think. Many surgeons will confirm that they feel most calm and relaxed while operating. Above all, to continue the operation list provided an excuse for silence.

Bailey returned to Denham and to Veta, and we shall never know what passed between them. A local general practitioner came to the hospital the next day expecting to find him there, and was told the news. He knew the Baileys slightly, and in the evening called at Fairlawn. telling the maid that he would only come up if they wanted to see him. He was there for two hours, and many years later, Veta recorded the comfort which this acquaintance had been able to afford them. They knew so many people and had so few friends.

But there was even worse to come

The woman whom Bailey had been operating on at Potters Bar at the time the news of his son's death arrived, had been given a blood transfusion. As was the practice in those days, Bailey had himself cross-matched the blood the evening before, using an elementary technique involving mixing red cells and plasma on a white tile. Knowing the complexity of the antigenic systems involved, it is extraordinary that fatal accidents did not happen every day as a result of this primitive procedure, but for whatever reasons they were quite unusual. Not so this time. The patient died following the operation, and it was suspected that the cause of death was a transfusion of blood which was incompatible. This was never proved, but the effect of this appalling double tragedy on a man such as Bailey, whose rough and abrupt behaviour sheltered a deep sense of self doubt, reinforced by his experiences in early life, was longlasting, and must have contributed to the grave problems which beset him in later years.

At the inquest held at Preston on 4 August, the Coroner recorded a verdict of death by misadventure. Railway employees testified that before the goods train had left Preston the doors were securely closed, and the court found that there was no evidence of neglect on the part of the LMS. Neither Veta nor her husband could bring themselves to attend, but sent a secretary, Lilian Jones, to report back to them. In later years, as the 11 June approached, Bailey would become withdrawn and irritable, and on the actual anniversary he would refuse to operate. Early on, he had insisted on removing all traces of his son's presence in the house, and was never heard to refer to him. Zina Fitzgerald felt that his emotion was rather one of remorse than grief, and this has been confirmed by others who knew him at the time. It was later recorded by one of his psychiatrists that he became permanently impotent following young Hamilton's death. As a widow, Veta developed many close friendships, but she never alluded to that dreadful day. A memorial still exists in the form of the Hamilton Bailey Prize, given to the best all round student in work and sport at Mill Hill (Figure 6.4).

The National Health Service

During the Second World War, many young men and women had time to reflect on the social systems which lay behind the conflict, and on the type of society to which they would return in the event of victory. Economists, philosophers and aspiring politicians, in spite of preoccupation with their own and their nation's survival, continued to examine the recent past and to suggest models of improvement. Crucial to this was the idea of universal provision of free health care, not only morally right but also cost effective since (it was argued) if everyone had good health, everyone would be more productive, hence the system would pay for itself. This was the central idea of the report produced by Lord Beveridge in 1944, resulting in a Government White Paper. Though virtuous, the idea was flawed, and we still live with its consequences.

The allies won the war. The Beveridge Report was adopted and formed the basis for the establishment of a National Health Service, which was adopted as policy by the incoming Labour Government in 1945. No one now doubts the altruism of this political choice, but at the time its effect on the voluntary charitable hospitals was disastrous. In 1945 the Royal Northern received nearly £11,000 in gifts and legacies and in the following year this fell to £370. The State was now in charge, and no one ever felt charitable towards the Inland Revenue. Costs continued to rise, and by 1947 the hospital was £250,000 in debt. Bailey had never been much interested in medical politics, but was not in principle opposed to the idea of a National Health Service. In fact he greatly admired the Danish system, which went some way towards state provision. However he abhorred bureaucratic control, and wrote an article in the *BMJ* in March 1948, later reissued in the *Journal of the International College of Surgeons*, which ended thus:

> *No, Sir, provided that scope is given for private enterprise, there is nothing fundamentally wrong with State medicine, but if you knew as well as I know the officials of the Ministry of Health, I am sure that every nerve in your body would cry out 'God forbid that they control me or my patients'.*

One particular result of the changes aroused his indignation. The designated Teaching Hospitals had been allowed to retain their boards of governors, through whom they had direct access to the Ministry of Health, and this he saw as unjustly favouring of the interests of these hospitals as against those such as the Royal Northern, which had no attachment to an undergraduate school. In 1945 Bailey was instrumental in founding an organisation with the rather clumsy title of 'The Association of Honorary Staffs of the Major Non-Undergraduate Teaching Hospitals', on the Council of which he represented the Royal Northern. Negotiations were taking place at that time with the Royal Free Hospital in Grays Inn Road, regarding training of medical students on the Northern site, but these broke down amid some acrimony, as the Northern sought equal status as a Teaching Hospital with the Royal Free, who had their own undergraduate school and quite different ideas as to their relative positions. In reply, the consultants at

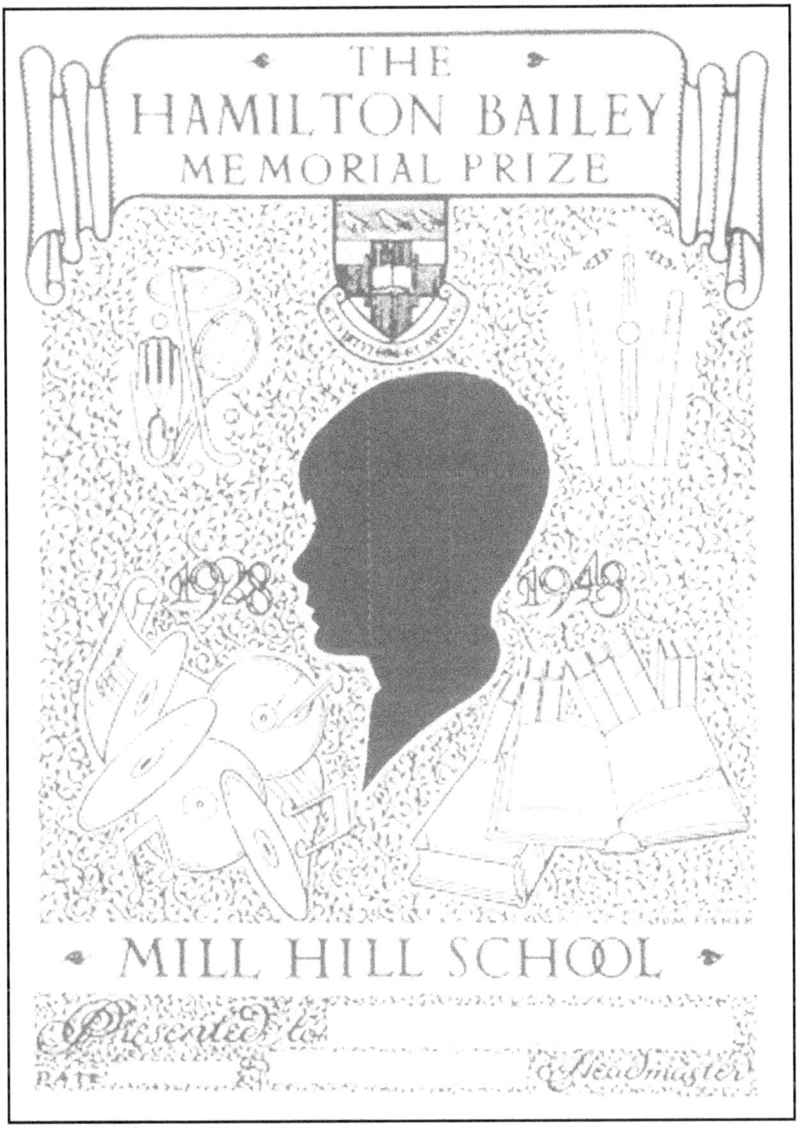

Figure 6.1: The prize in memory of young Hamilton

the Northern refused to continue teaching the students. This seems a rather petulant and short-sighted decision, though of course students still continued to arrive from St Bartholomew's and The Middlesex. However Bailey vigorously and successfully opposed what he saw as an unjust distribution of beds between the two sites, and fought a campaign to ensure that supplies of the new miracle drug penicillin should be allocated to the Northern. He persuaded a local MP, Sir Graham Hill, to raise the question in Parliament, but this was vetoed by the Medical Committee who felt that it was inappropriate for them to become involved politically. The other contentious issue was whether the specialist hospitals, such as the Sick Childrens' Hospital in Great Ormond Street and St Mark's Hospital for colorectal disorders, should be admitted to the Association, and this again was opposed by Bailey, somewhat short-sightedly, in fact, as they would have proved powerful allies, with a great deal of charitable support. Together with McNeill Love (who in 1945 was elected to the Council of the Royal College of Surgeons, probably somewhat to Bailey's chagrin) he then proposed the formation of a joint Postgraduate Medical School with the Prince of Wales Hospital, Tottenham, but this rather unlikely scheme made little progress.

The 'appointed day' was 5 July 1948, on which the local authority and voluntary hospitals were taken over by the NHS, and although a somewhat nostalgic occasion the change nonetheless brought relief from what was quickly becoming an impossible financial situation. The Northern came under the jurisdiction of the North West Metropolitan Regional Hospital Board, and the old Board of Management with its Chairman, was dissolved. Royal presidency came to an end, although the Duke of Gloucester agreed to continue his association with the hospital by becoming its Patron. The Royal Northern became part of a group of ten hospitals in the new region, and lost its autonomy to a body known as the Northern Group Hospital Management Committee, but as the hospital had formed the hub of just such a group for a number of years, these apparently radical changes had comparatively little effect on its sphere of influence. Emergency cases and outpatients continued to arrive, junior doctors and students were still taught, and the daughters of nurses who had trained at the Northern maintained recruitment to the preliminary training school. Under the National Health Service St David's Wing went on receiving private patients and provided useful income for the hospital, although the number of beds was reduced.

Decline and Fall

The committee minutes and operation books over the later war years show that during this time Bailey was more and more restricting himself (or being restricted) to comparatively minor operations such hernia repair and removal of haemorrhoids. The number of major abdominal explorations became very limited, and it has to be asked why this was the case. Was it that the practice of the Royal Northern Hospital in major surgery was going elsewhere, or was it simply that because of declining powers and increasing personal problems he was deliberately scaling down his operation lists? One can only speculate, but there is no reason to suppose that the number of those requiring major surgery was in any way diminishing in North London at that time. Another feature of his surgical practice, which was later commented on by Allan Clain, is his liking for 'staged' operations, and there are many references to 'first stage' gastrectomy and 'second stage' prostatectomy. Clain observed that as the years went by Bailey's decisiveness began to falter, not only in the operating theatre but also in his personal life, and he preferred instinctively to delay activities and carry them out in successive stages, whether or not this was always appropriate.

In the middle and later 1940s, the inherited mental problems began to surface, although at first quite gradually. It was clear that the frenetic activity of the 1930s involving eight hours a day, six or seven days a week in the operating theatre, with every evening being taken up with writing and editing, could no longer be sustained. The war years had been exhausting, and the prospect of radical social change and a threat to the way of life built up with such difficulty, became an obsession. As his opinion became less sought and the clinical pace slackened, with a corresponding demand on administrative skills which he had never really developed, Bailey grew increasingly irritable and unpredictable, and eventually began to miss appointments and make simple diagnostic mistakes. In 1946 while in Canada he made a speech deploring the decline in standards of British nursing who, he said, 'now deserted their patients for enjoyment...' The Royal Northern nurses protested furiously to the Chairman of the Medical Committee, who was forced to apologise. No formal reprimand was made to Bailey on his return, but almost certainly the Chairman would have had some very frank words in private.

Next, his performance in the operating theatre, always open to criticism, began to deteriorate alarmingly. The junior staff grew restive, and complaints began to come in to managers and colleagues. In early 1947 it was recorded that a pack was left in the abdomen of one of his patients. Today, of course, such an incident would have been made public and an enquiry and action for negligence would have certainly followed, but the trusting and uncomplaining view which the general public took of doctors in those days enabled the hospital authorities to keep the matter quiet. Veta covered up for him in every possible way, but before very long it was plain to all that something was seriously wrong, and that Bailey was no longer a safe surgeon. Referrals from general practitioners began to fall off, and rumours began to circulate. The manifestations of severe mental disturbance became more frequent, and caused problems with Veta and her family, and increasing anxiety and concern amongst his professional colleagues. There was an outburst of uncontrollable rage in the operating theatre at St Vincent's clinic, tactfully hushed up by the faithful Sister Pauline. Bailey was at first reluctant to concede that anything was wrong, and to accept the need for help, but eventually Dr Lindsay Neustatter, his psychiatric colleague at the Northern, was called in and made a diagnosis of 'impending mania'. The records over the next months are fragmentary, but it is clear that he was taking long and frequent periods of sick leave, though some of these were spent in writing books or attending foreign conferences. He was offered the Presidency of the International College of Surgeons, which in former times would have delighted him, but by now he was too ill to accept it.

A little time before, frustrated and unhappy, Bailey had applied for the Chair of Surgery at the University of Cape Town, on the retirement of Professor Charles Saint. Saint had gained fame by drawing attention to the frequent association between hiatus hernia, gallstones and diverticula of the colon, the so-called 'Saint's Triad', a type of concept which confused coincidence with causation, quite unsupported by figures, but which had great appeal to surgeons of Bailey's generation. Bearing in mind his international reputation as an author and teacher, Bailey's request to be considered for the South African chair was probably not unrealistic, but in fact he was never a serious candidate. Alan Clain, who knew the individuals involved in the decision, feels that this was because of his poor reputation as a practical surgeon, but it is at least possible that rumours of unreliable behaviour and mental instability had already reached Cape Town. What is curious (but perhaps typical of Bailey's naïve and somewhat arrogant approach) is that he took the trouble to report this unsuccessful application to the Medical Staff Committee at the Royal Northern, who recorded it in their minutes of November 1946. He did not attend that particular meeting, but throughout the next year and a half his presence there, which had previously been rather spasmodic (he was never proposed as its Chairman), became rather more regular, apart from the periods of sick leave, and he continued to attend right up to June 1948. It was no coincidence that this paralleled a corresponding decrease in his contact with patients

He did however continue to write, to see private patients and even occasionally to carry out simple operations at St Vincent's Clinic and St David's Wing. These sessions were extremely worrying occasions for the anaesthetic and nursing staff, as Bailey's hands shook and he found it almost impossible to concentrate.

At this point, he became more dependent on the nurses who understood his strengths and weaknesses, and continued to support him. Sister Wheable had been with him in the outpatient clinics, wards and operating theatres. 'I loved him', she said. 'He was grand to work with...He was efficient; he couldn't stand idiots; he liked everything to go with a swing. He was very kind to his patients and they liked him. They knew where they stood with him...'. Claire Rayner, who as a young student nurse at the Royal Northern from time to time assisted him in the operating theatre, remembers how the faithful Sister Wheable gently guided Bailey through the steps of a hernia repair.

Looking back, it seems quite incomprehensible that responsible people who were aware of the problem stood by while patients were put at risk at the hands of a dangerously sick man, but of course the perspectives at that time were very different. Loyalty to the chief and to the institution was everything. The authority of a consultant surgeon was virtually unchallengeable, except by senior colleagues, and they probably knew little of what was going on. Surgeons in the same hospital seldom visit each others' operating theatres. Bernard Shaw observed that all professions are conspiracies against the laity, and here was a clear example. This conspiracy persisted for many years, but public opinion has now changed, and the result has been a backlash of resentment and distrust of consultant physicians and surgeons, whose authority and status has dwindled and whose movements are controlled by the managers and clerks they once despised.

As things grew worse, Neustatter called in various psychiatric colleagues, but the one he and Veta seems to have had most confidence in was Dr Desmond Curran, later Professor of Psychiatry at St George's' Hospital and President of the Royal College. On 12 August 1948 Neustatter admitted Bailey to Napsbury Hospital at St Albans, with a diagnosis of 'manic depressive insanity' where he underwent courses of sedation alternating with the passage of high voltage shocks through the brain, known as electroconvulsive therapy (ECT). He left after a few weeks but soon afterwards relapsed and was readmitted. Once again he returned home, but grew worse, and Neustatter called in Desmond Curran who recorded that he was depressed and paranoid, and felt that the outlook was bad. His behaviour became more and disorganised, and early in 1949 Curran transferred him under an urgency order to St Andrew's Hospital, Northampton, a private mental facility, with the diagnosis of acute manic excitement, where he underwent a further 22 courses of ECT, anaesthetised with pentothal and curare. This was followed by a course of 'continuous narcosis', which involved prolonged periods of drug-induced unconsciousness, a treatment favoured by his colleague Neustatter. However this also was ineffective and he relapsed into a depressive state with paranoid misinterpretations. The Medical Committee minutes for March 1949 recommend that he be granted a 'further period of six months' sick leave with effect from the 1st April'. Immediately following this, on Bailey's insistence and against medical advice, Veta removed him from hospital care.

At the meeting of the Medical Committee at the Royal Northern Hospital on 27 September 1949 a letter from Bailey was read out announcing that he had come to the conclusion that he must give up active surgical work as a result of his long and severe illness. It was unanimously decided that a letter be written to Mr Bailey and signed by the Senior Surgeon, the Chairman and the Honorary Secretary of the Committee, expressing the regret of the Committee. In retrospect, this perfunctory message of sympathy seems dismally inadequate. His colleagues clearly had no inkling that one of their members had a reputation that would far outlive them.

Bailey never went back. The Royal Northern Hospital continued to flourish for many years after his departure, and attracted a distinguished medical staff, most of whom held parallel appointments at the major teaching hospitals. However, as described in Chapter 4, the decision to locate the main acute facilities for the Islington population in Highgate led to a general decline, and the final closure in 1992.

Chapter 7
THE MENTAL NEMESIS

Worthing

In April 1949, at his own insistence and with Veta's less than wholehearted consent, Bailey left St Andrew's, accompanied by a private nurse, and went to stay with his mother's sister Edith in Worthing. Aunt Edith had always been fond of him, as he was of her, and in contrast to Margaret, she was a model of kindness and stability. She had retired from hospital work, and ran a small private nursing home at 25a Church Walk, under the supervision of a local general practitioner, Dr Wilshaw. Edith gave notice to her paying tenant and made over the whole top floor of her house to Hamilton and Veta, and Dr Curran arranged for Dr Edward Charlton, the deputy superintendent of Graylingwell Mental Hospital near Chichester, to see him at home. Treatment was continued with sedation, and in early 1950 he underwent a course of insulin coma, in a private nursing home, again under the supervision of Dr Neustatter. To induce hypoglycaemic fits in an elderly man would seem to invite calamity, and indeed this form of treatment probably did claim some deaths (much, it must be admitted, as had surgery as practised by Bailey and others), but his strong frame was able to withstand such onslaughts, which in the event proved quite as ineffective as had all the previous courses of ECT. He remained constantly depressed, frightened and unable to sleep. Life at Church Walk must at times have been intolerable. It was like having a disturbed and noisy child in the house, but in this case the child was six foot tall and used to exercising authority. Amazingly, Bailey was able in spite of this to continue revising his books, although (as had always been the case) much of the work was done by Veta. New editions of *Short Practice* came out in 1948 and 1952, of *Physical Signs* in 1949 and 1954, and Allan Clain also visited him at this time, in connection with these books and with *Pye's Surgical Handicraft*. All of this involved writing and receiving letters from colleagues, reproducing photographs, trips to London to the libraries of the Royal Society of Medicine and the Royal College of Surgeons, and constant docketing and filing of new material. The Rolls Royce had been stored away and replaced by something smaller. Bailey who had neither enjoyed driving nor been very good at it, was by now quite unfit to be in charge of a car, so that once again the responsibility for the arrangements fell upon Veta. Sometimes they went by train, sometimes Veta drove, but often Bailey was so disturbed that it was impossible for him to get out of the house.

Matters came to a head in the summer of 1951, when the devoted and selfless Edith finally lost her patience, and asked her nephew and his wife to leave the upstairs flat. They transferred to the nearby Downlands Hotel, but Bailey became noisy and uncontrollable, roamed through the public rooms in the middle of the night, offended guests in the rather prim and decorous dining room, and within a few weeks the manager insisted that they went elsewhere.

Chichester

The next move was to the house of Veta's sister Dagmar, who had married an insurance agent called MacHattie and lived at Hazel House in the attractive village of Elsted near Midhurst, where they had an orchard and a smallholding. Unlike Veta, who had no particular interest in her ancestry, and was more concerned with her husband's professional advancement, Dagmar was proud of her Swedish origins and kept in touch with relations there. The sisters had always been close, and Dagmar had been a frequent visitor to the house in Totteridge, had been very fond of young Hamilton, and was pleased to be of help in the present crisis. At first, this new refuge seemed to be a success, and the MacHatties were tolerant of occasional outbursts and explosions, and respectful of Veta's literary activities. But Bailey's mental pain did not improve, and he became more and more restless and difficult to cope with. In desperation, Veta wrote to Desmond Curran, who in turn communicated with Dr Jonathan Carse, the medical superintendent of Graylingwell Hospital, asking for his help over poor 'Hamilton Bailey'. Dr Carse made arrangements for a further course of ECT to be administered at The Acre, Boundary Road, which was the Worthing annexe of Graylingwell. The first treatment was due to be given on 18 July 1951, but probably never took place because of Veta's objections. On 11 September 1951 things became so bad that Dagmar telephoned Dr Desmond Hanbury, who was not only a general practitioner in Midhurst but also held a psychiatric appointment at Graylingwell, with a view to relieving the family of their burden by 'certifying' her brother in law, which would mean that he would be consigned to a mental hospital and would lose his civil rights. The certificate was in two stages, an Urgency Order designed to deal with a crisis, and a longer permanent certificate granted as a result of more leisured psychiatric assessment. The Urgency Order, dated 11 September 1951 and signed by Dr Hanbury, gives the reason for Bailey's incarceration as 'he is suffering from manic depressive psychosis and is not in a fit state to look after himself nor can he be adequately cared for in his present situation' (Figure 7.1). Dr Hanbury formed his conclusion on the following grounds.

He talks incessantly, says that he is drugged into his present state. He constantly asks to telephone a number of doctors saying they will be able to cure him. His conversation constantly changes to new unrelated subjects. He frequently says he is 'acting' because of mental disease. He is always asking for proof and for verification of simple occurrences. He says his wife is responsible for his present illness. He is getting careless in his personal hygiene although he has always been most particular in this respect.

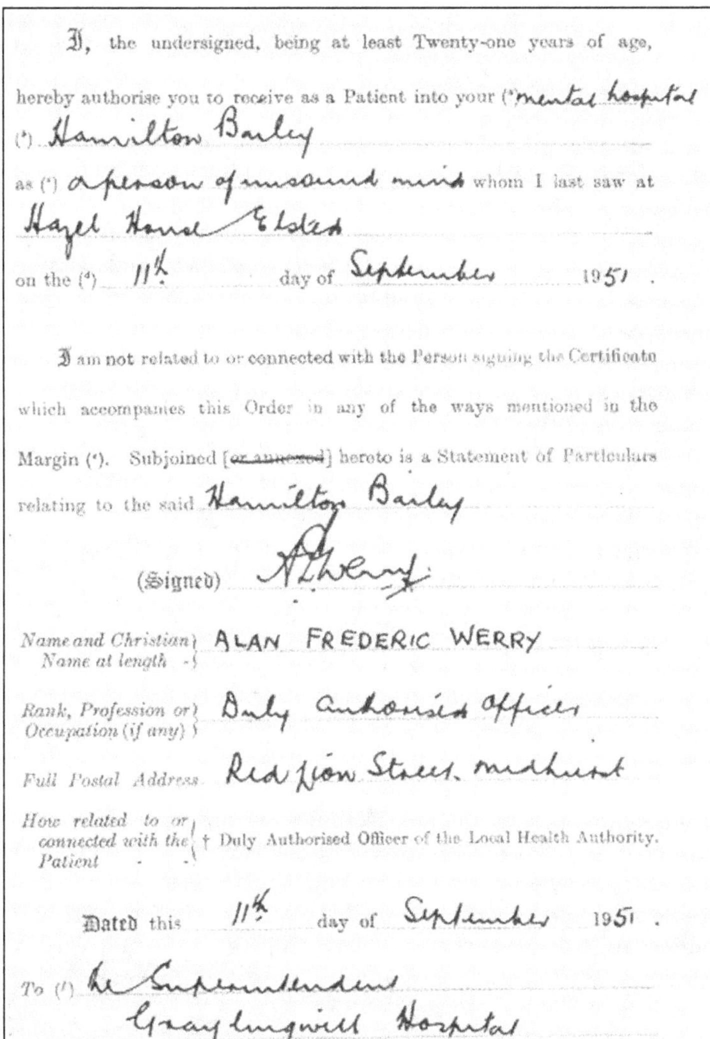

I, the undersigned, being at least Twenty-one years of age, hereby authorise you to receive as a Patient into your ( ) mental hospital

( ) Hamilton Barley

as ( ) a person of unsound mind whom I last saw at Hazel House Elsted

on the ( ) 11th day of September 1951.

I am not related to or connected with the Person signing the Certificate which accompanies this Order in any of the ways mentioned in the Margin ( ). Subjoined [~~or annexed~~] hereto is a Statement of Particulars relating to the said Hamilton Barley

(Signed) A L Werry

Name and Christian Name at length: ALAN FREDERIC WERRY

Rank, Profession or Occupation (if any): Duly authorised Officer

Full Postal Address: Red Lion Street, Midhurst

How related to or connected with the Patient: † Duly Authorised Officer of the Local Health Authority.

Dated this 11th day of September 1951.

To ( ) The Superintendent
Graylingwell Hospital

Figure 7.1: The Urgency Order

So once again Bailey arrived at the front door of a hospital, but this time not in a Rolls Royce but in a Sussex County ambulance. He was admitted under the care of the Consultant Psychiatrist, Dr David Rice, with the diagnosis of 'mania', and the admission note records that he was 'overactive, overtalkative, hostile, aggressive, writing continuously'. Bailey's condition when he arrived at the place that was to be his home for the next three years was truly pitiful. This large, dominant, commanding man had been reduced to an introspective, self-regarding wreck, barely capable of looking after his own physical needs. To make matters worse, finding himself in the familiar environment of a hospital, he at once assumed an authoritative role and made pathetic efforts to take control of events, and the patient and understanding attitude of the doctors and nurses recorded in the notes at that time, who had to put up with much arrogance and insult, is impressive. His habit of cross-questioning everyone who came to see him, dictating instructions and giving inappropriate and confused commands, must have been quite intolerable.

At this supremely difficult moment, Veta herself was admitted to hospital. For some time her nights had been disturbed by severe attacks of pain under her ribs, and an X-ray had shown gallstones. Before he was certified, Hamilton had contacted his surgical colleague Harold Dodd, and had arranged for Veta to go into St Vincent's Clinic. He insisted on organising all details of his wife's admission, and besides choosing and instructing the anaesthetist, gave precise directions as to the way the surgery should be carried out, and how the abdominal wall should be closed, including the number and type of stitches to be used. It was typical of him that, although a part of his brain was disintegrating, the old reflexes still functioned and, although now a certified patient in a mental hospital, he was able to convince the nursing staff at St Vincent's, in particular Sister Pauline, that he was still in command of the situation, and that his instructions should be obeyed. The day after Hamilton's admission, Veta underwent her operation.

Graylingwell

The first thing that Bailey did on his admission to Graylingwell (Figure 7.2) was to telephone Aunt Edith and ask her to send a car to take him home. When she explained that this was not possible, he said 'I will never speak to you again'. 'And I don't suppose he will', was Edith's philosophical reply. Of course, her reaction was right. Her nephew was in no condition to go anywhere,and his mental state became much worse over the next few days. One of his nurses, John Seals, reported:

> *He steals things from the rooms etc. and throws them out of the corridors. He has boasted of having tried to commit suicide. He accuses his wife of being responsible for his present illness. He constantly asks to see further doctors. He wants to 'phone and go shopping in the middle of the night. He hoards medicines and clothing*

belonging to other people and will only give them back on 'special terms'. He is constantly writing down other peoples' statements and asking them to be signed to make them 'evidence'. He talks constantly, changing the subject very frequently. He will not believe his wife is in hospital although she went there yesterday. He says he has tried to commit suicide and has handed over his razor blades in case he wants to try again. He changes frequently in regarding people as friends and enemies.

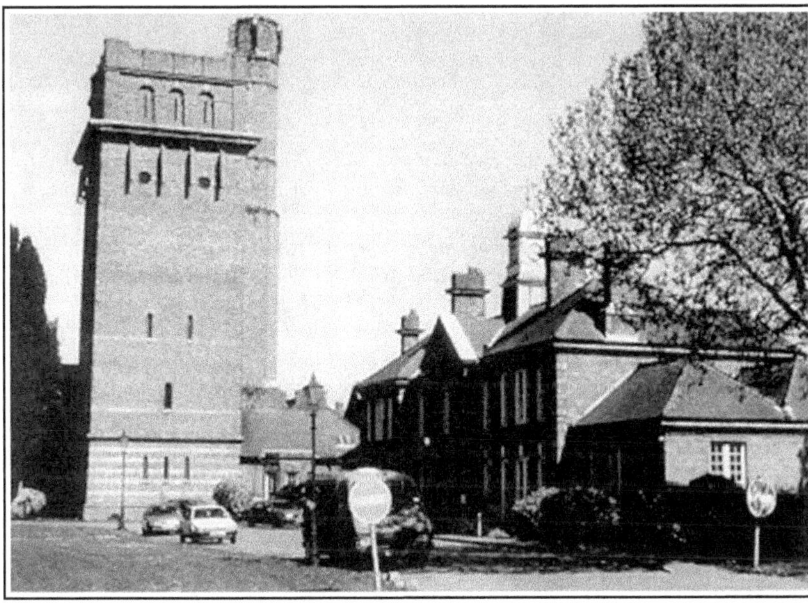

Figure 7.2: Graylingwell

The record from there onwards is one of despair and degradation, with alternating moods of fatuous optimism and exaggerated gratitude. There were moments of insight. Thus on 22 September 1951, Bailey wrote:

How can I ever be a surgeon again? Mental illness is no more shameful than a G.U., but all my friends abandon me. The psychiatric patient is never believed

But a few days later:

Dear Dr Carse. How wonderful it is to be under a medical superintendent who has my case so much at heart! I am sure I have turned the corner. Please thank all who are assisting in my recovery.

Yours very sincerely, HB.

And yet at the same time the medical notes record that he was untidy, stained and with two to four days beard, demanding to see solicitors, full of complaints, and repeatedly telephoning doctors and lawyers. On 30 September it is recorded that 'the doctors should come when I send for them'. These summons were not obeyed.

In spite of recovering from a painful operation, Veta wrote to him every day. Bailey either tore up the letters or threw them into a corner, whence they were retrieved by the nurses, and included in the clinical record. The messages are full of tender support, tinged with the gentlest of reproaches. Thus:

St Vincents Clinic
Wednesday

My dearest
I was bitterly disappointed to find that you had not written to me again today. I was sure that if you knew how much I longed to hear from you, you would do so.

Just as you must be worrying about me, so you must realise that I worry about you. I telephoned the hospital last night, and was much cheered to learn that they are pleased with your progress.

I had my stitches out yesterday, and dressed and went into the garden. I felt very weak, but at least it is a start. How I wish that the cholecystectomy had been performed through a tramsvrese (sic) *incision!*

Now all we both have to do is to concentrate on getting better as quickly as possible, and being together again. I cannot tell you how desperately I miss you and long to be with you...

Write to me my darling. It would cheer me up so much.

A few days later:

St Vincent's Clinic
Sunday

My darling
As you have not taken any notice of my pleas for you to write me a letter, I have come to the conclusion that perhaps you are not even opening my letters - because I cannot believe that if you knew how anxious I was to hear from you, you would not write to me.

I am writing to let you know my future movements. Harold Dodd says that he wants me to have a full month of convalescence before returning to any work, domestic or otherwise. On Tuesday next Mr Clain is going to run me down to the Southdowns Hotel, and I shall stay there for a week to get stronger. My wounds have not quite healed yet, and I shall have to go rather carefully. At the end of that time I shall get in touch with you again, to see if you want me to come to you. If, in the present state of your illness you feel that you would rather not see me and would like to concentrate on getting better yourself, I shall quite understand, my dearest. Always remember that I always wanted what is best for you.

I have just sent off the corrected proofs of the last two galley proofs of your section of Short Practice, and when I get back I will get on with the first three chapters of Surgery for Nurses. Indeed, it will give the publishers something to be getting on with.

All my love darling,
forever,
your Veta.

It is not known whether Hamilton read this letter. However, in a letter to the Medical Superintendent on 20 October 1951 he wrote:

my wife was threatening to leave me and take a job in Ireland. Tremendous effort of will to open those letters. The long clinical training has permitted me to read peoples' faces. After 25 years I can read my wife's face like a book. She has not carried out the instructions re appointment with Moss (the Dentist). I will therefore be (I hope) a MODEL certified lunatic patient.

The next day he wrote to his Worthing GP, Dr Eddison,

Doubtless in sympathy with Aunt Edith you have roundly condemned me for not writing to Veta when she was in St Vincent's, the arrangements for which you will doubtless recall you left entirely to me.

Be that as it may in 14 days please ring Park 8391 and ask for Sister Margaret, get this Christian woman's impartial judgement. Particularly ask Sr. Margaret if I have ever been selfish. She has known me much longer than you.

Am not at all satisfied with Veta's genitocrural neuritis - will write to to you and Aunt Edith about this within 3 days. If they post the letter see later you will get my views for what they are worth. But I do know her case inside out - who could no [sic] *more?*

It is unlikely that they showed Veta this particular letter, and perhaps it is just as well that she did not see it. At this time, nobody wrote to Bailey except his wife, and he could not, or would not, respond to her. He wrote continuously to other people, and although the messages were often illogical and out of place, they were written in a firm and clear hand. Thus on 17 October 1951 he writes

One calendar month after my admission. Where are my letters to Dr Wilshaw and Dagmar?

On 19 October 1951 he wrote to his consultant Dr Rice (enclosing a copy to Dr Desmond Curran) saying 'ECT is so old-fashioned'. At the same time he demanded to be seen by Lord Moran (described as President of the Royal College of Surgeons but who was in fact a physician - a most unusual slip for Bailey to make), Sir Russell Brain (an eminent neurologist) and once again Dr Lindsey Neustatter.

Meanwhile, the nurses' records give a very different impression from that of a calm professional writing letters in a quiet corner. Rather they rather describe a dishevelled elderly man with several days' growth of beard, often abusive, arrogant, recalcitrant to treatment, throwing his possessions about and refusing to dress himself, at times smearing his room with excrement. He was agressive towards the other patients on the ward, some of whom were very severely disturbed, but all of whom regarded their fellow inmate as 'totally mad'. He would store rubbish up in small lockers, hide his clothes, and occasionally throw his dentures out of the window into the garden, and laugh as the staff went down to pick them up.

As soon as Veta got out of hospital, she started to visit, to bring her husband small comforts, and to have regular discussions with Dr Carse and David Rice. These were not always easy. At one particularly difficult time Rice records 'she takes some part in her husband's antics. She wrote regularly but seldom received a reply. Thus on 6 November she wrote:

My dearest Hamilton

I stayed at Elsted overnight, and only received your letter when I got back last night. I was overjoyed to get it - especially when I had left you the previous day in such an unhappy frame of mind. Your letter was much more loving to me, and I have gained much comfort from it.

I am glad that you have decided to keep on with the Whitmore and Bailey cigarettes; as you say it would be a pity to give them up after all those years. I will also keep on the whisky, as you wish me to do so. I have not been tempted to do this, as now that I do not need extra meat for you, I have no object in ordering it. However, I think you are wise and should keep on this connection, and I will build up a supply, as you may need it for presents later.

Although you did not look into the things I brought you on Sunday, I hope you have done so by now. I have tried hard to put everything you have asked for (contrary to what you believed I did the whole of the shopping myself, and it took me three days to find everything I brought). Will you let me know if the pants I have ordered for you...fit you now. If they do I will have more done to the same size...I shall not come to see you on Wednesday (the day you get this letter, I hope) because I felt very strongly on Sunday that my visits tend to upset you - and that is the last thing I wish to do. Please believe me, darling, that I have no wish to either part or have a divorce. The desire that we should be parted emanates entirely from you. It hurts me very much that after all these years of close friendship and co-operation you should wish it to cease, just at the time when we should be beginning to enjoy a well-earned rest from all our very great labours. All I want at the moment is for you to get better, and for us to live together in happiness.

Aunt Edith tells me that you have given her notice as from 31st December this year. Where would you like us to live? Had you thought that I must have a home while you are in hospital? If you have any desire to live elsewhere let me know, and I will try and find accommodation, but you know it is very difficult to find a suitable and reasonable place these days. With all my love.

p.s. I thought you might like to see the enclosed receipt. On 2nd November I paid a further £10.00 into your account at the hospital. I am told that you draw out about £2.00 a week of this. I will see that you are never left without money in the account, and you can draw as you wish.

These letters were not often answered: many of then were torn up or left unopened. During all this time, Bailey was constantly smoking, initially using some 70 'Woodbines' each day, and subsequently rolling his own cigarettes. (Woodbines together with 'Player's Weights', were the cheapest and least regarded brand of British cigarette. They had been charitably distributed during the First World War by the famous Army Chaplain, the Reverend W. Studdert Kennedy, who was known as 'Woodbine Willie'. In his days at Fairlawn or Harley Street, Hamilton Bailey would never have considered smoking a Woodbine. Gentlemen smoked Players' Navy Cut, Gold Flake or Three Castles. Was this a sort of ironic throwback to the days in Bristol, where his prospects had so much depended on Wills money? Unlike many of his colleagues, however, Bailey had never been a heavy drinker. An occasional glass of whisky in the evening was all that he ever required, and Veta's letter makes clear that the only use he made of the bottles she sent him was as gifts to his fellow patients.

As the months went on, he became more and more disruptive, attacking the nursing staff and other patients, so that eventually he was locked into a single room. Nonetheless, he was gently and understandingly treated. The daily notes recorded by Nurses Miller, Hyde, Dicker, Seal and Morrier (all of them men) are a model of forbearance and compassion. Bearing in mind that Graylingwell was a public mental hospital in a country district, and that this was only a few years after the end of the Second World War, when economic circumstances were not easy, the sympathetic attitude of the staff towards this extremely demanding and agressive patient commands admiration.

Throughout 1951 and 1952 treatment was continued with sedation and ECT at intervals. Early in 1952 it seems that the psychiatrists were inclining towards a diagnosis of schizophrenia, and the question of a prefrontal leucotomy was raised. This operation involves cutting the nerve fibres between the main part of the cerebral cortex and the portion of the brain lying immediately above the eyes. It had been shown to calm violent apes, and had been developed in human patients by the Portuguese neurosurgeon Egas Moniz, who had been given a Nobel Prize for his work, having proved its effectiveness in reducing manic patients to some degree of docility. Veta strongly resisted the suggested leucotomy, and her fears were reinforced by the fact that Bailey's long-forgotten schizophrenic sister May had undergone the operation at Haywards Heath many years previously, and now aged 53 was totally disorientated.

The picture during 1952 is one of continuing deterioration. Nurse Hide records on 20 July 1952,

> *Will steal anything from the other patients he sees lying around. Accuses patients of having things belonging to him and investigates by putting hands in their pockets, this leads to arguments and struggles. Continuously asks foolish questions and demands to see MO's all day. Throws his dentures about the ward and when in exercise garden will raise ward windows and throw stones into them. Then his shoes followed by his dentures again. If they are put away he becomes a perfect pest asking for them. Continues to smoke more than 50 cigarettes per day and no doubt is relieved of some by patients. Requires undressing at bedtime and has to be dressed in the morning. Will not help himself. Certainly a ward problem.*

There followed by a period of comparative tranquillity, but the nurses and doctors found no cause for optimism. In September 1952 Dr Rice reports 'deteriorated. Flat. Affectless. The pathetic shadow and shell of a previously warm, whole-hearted individual full of drive and purpose'. And a little later 'Not much change. Quieter. Content to sit in chair and do nothing if left - no longer troublesome or interfering. Abusive to his wife when she visits and destructive to his clothing'.

Repeated pressure was put on Veta to agree to the leucotomy, and eventually it was explained to her that although it might not benefit her husband, it was required as a controlling measure, to prevent him victimising the other patients and the nurses, many of whom were smaller and weaker. During the whole of this time, in spite of his visible deterioration, Bailey continued to write. He wrote ceaselessly, letters to doctors, to lawyers and to politicians, reminiscences, surgical anecdotes and aphorisms, and all with a firm and logical hand. He had an amazing capacity for remembering the names, titles, degrees and appointments of colleagues all over the UK and indeed the world, to whom he addressed pathetic and at times arrogant messages. There is no record of any reply.

On 10 October 1952 Veta persuaded Desmond Curran to come once more to see his old patient. Bailey could not, or would not, recognise him: 'that Dr Curran is not the Dr Curran I know'. Curran agreed with Rice that the prognosis was hopeless, and that no treatment was possible. In view of Bailey's previous personality and episodes of mania he took the view that leucotomy might make things worse. Curran's visit was followed by a resumption of noisy and disruptive behaviour (accompanied by delusions and outbursts of paranoia). However, his physical condition remained surprisingly good and at a routine physical examination in March 1953 it was recorded that he was in excellent shape, and that his weight was going up. There was no improvement during the remainder of that year, and he is repeatedly recorded as being 'aggressive, untidy, resentful of attention and unreliable in mood. He makes constant accusations against the other patients and the staff, and frequently writes letters to professional colleagues, which do not usually receive any replies'.

In desperation, Dr Rice and his colleagues finally decided that, regardless of expert opinion, a leucotomy was unavoidable, if only in the interests of the other patients. Under enormous pressure Veta finally gave her consent to the operation on 29 September 1953, and arrangements were put in hand for Wiley McKissock, an eminent neurosurgeon from St George's Hospital in London, to come down to Chichester and carry it out. Everyone, except perhaps Veta, agreed that Hamilton Bailey would never leave hospital, and that by whatever means he must be calmed down, in the interests of himself and of the fellow sufferers with whom he would spend the rest of his life

In the meantime, Veta had been forced to sell Denham and to move into something smaller. She chose a flat in Worthing, near to Edith, and within reach of Chichester. The house in Totteridge housed a collection of 4000 books. Some of them had been bought by her husband, but many were signed copies from colleagues all over the world. Also included of course were all of the editions of Bailey's own works, to which she had contributed so much. The aftermath of a world war was not the best time to sell a medical library, and Veta received much less than its ultimate market value.

During his three years stay at Graylingwell, Veta's belief in her husband's inner normality had never faltered. In the face of his physical and mental disintegration, his callous rejection of her help, affection and loyalty, his abuse and false accusations, his anger, resentment and total self absorption, his suspicion of her motives, it would have been easy to decide that this was not the man she had married, and that he had in some way been taken over by an alien force, so that she owed him no further allegiance. One could not blame any woman for reacting in that way, but Veta took the opposite view. Throughout, she maintained that her own Hamilton was still there, although afflicted by a terrible illness, and that if only the right treatment could be found, the true man would once more emerge. Perhaps her ultimate acceptance of the leucotomy represented a slight wavering of faith but, as it turned out, her reward was at hand.

One of the Registrars on Dr Rice's team was a young Australian, Dr David Moore. He told his Consultant about a new drug, lithium carbonate, which was being used in Sydney for the treatment of mania, and suggested that it should be tried in Bailey's case, in the hope of avoiding a leucotomy. Rice was intelligent and modest enough to accept advice from a junior colleague - something which Bailey himself would never have been able to do. On 7 October 1953 treatment was started with 600mg three times a day of lithium carbonate, to be given each day from Monday to Saturday, while at the same time the sedation was discontinued. Three days later the nursing notes report him as being 'quieter', and on 13th as 'much less hostile'. Dr Rice thereupon reversed his policy and decided that in view of even this slight degree of progress, the leucotomy operation should be held over.

The improvement continued. On 28 October it was recorded that his attitude to the staff had markedly improved. He was no longer hostile, said please and thank you, and did not pour obscene abuse at them. He was visited by his aunt and sat and spoke quietly with her. He was slightly tidier. During November, however, there was a relapse, and on learning of this Veta decided to spend Christmas in Liverpool to be with her by now aged and infirm parents.

Something quite extraordinary then happened. Bailey had not written to his wife for nearly three years, but on Christmas Eve 1953 he wrote a letter to her asking her to take him out, for he could not understand why, having completely recovered, he was still detained in hospital. The letter was sent to the flat in Worthing, while Veta was still in the North. Meanwhile, at Graylingwell, Christmas Day proved to be a problem. It was customary for the staff to join in the festivities with the patients, and to share a drink and a meal with them, but this was too much for Bailey to contemplate. He had suddenly became aware of his behaviour over the previous two years, and was bitterly ashamed, and feared that his appearance might be made an occasion for ridicule. During the staff visit he disappeared, and was found at the end of the garden some time later. He at first refused to come back and encounter his mentors/tormentors, but at the last minute reason prevailed, and he asked to see the doctors and nurses and thank them personally for their kindness and attention.

The recovery continued. By 27 December he was recorded as being rational, clear and tidy, and his habit of hoarding rubbish and storing away rotting material, seemed to have been abandoned. The following day, Dr Rice felt able to transfer him to an open ward, so that he could associate freely with fellow patients.

On 28 December he requested a special interview with Dr Rice, who recorded that:

> *He spoke reasonably and sensibly to me. Very anxious to leave the hospital etc. Now he has written to his wife and his aunt saying that he is shortly for discharge. When seen about this he is reasonably sensible - realises that the idea was premature. However he is clean, tidy and polite, has taken the trouble to make himself presentable, sits quietly and talks well. He would appreciate a chance to show himself as improving and must certainly have it.*

Following this he was transferred to an open ward, and when offered occupational therapy decided that he would prefer to work on his books. On 30 December the lithium was reduced to one tablet daily, and two weeks later he is again recorded as being clean, tidy and polite. By that time, Veta had returned to Worthing, where among a pile of Christmas cards she found, to her amazement, an envelope written in the clear, familiar, unmistakable hand of her husband, the first letter that he had written to her for two years. She immediately went back to Graylingwell, and found a Hamilton, who, if not actually affectionate, nonetheless recognised and greeted her. Dr Rice agreed that she should now visit regularly and take him out for drives in the countryside. He went on to say:

He is enjoying outings with his wife on each visiting day and is slightly anxious about leaving, and his capacity to recover monetary control of his affairs. He is certainly maintaining his fantastic improvement - one wonders if this can last. There is no evidence of depressive ideation. Lithium stopped from today.

However, there were some reservations. On 14 January Rice wrote:

Interviewed at some length following long interview with wife yesterday. She wishes to take him out on Sunday next 17th January for a holiday with a view to discharge. He has gained no insight whatever. He attributes his long illness to the environment, to the ECT, to everything possible other than illness. Thinks he would have behaved better if environment had been more congenial, if this that or the other. He is v. careful of what he says, avoids direct answers to any questions, brings in many irrelevant things to account fore his behaviour etc. He is anxious about discharge, tries to get exact details etc. and plans to go back to practice and to his hospital appointments as well as to his writing. Is planning a trip to America etc. He asks for details in relation to events of his illness but counters every item mentioned with what to him must be adequate reasons. Pleasant polite and co operative - memory is excellent. Judgement and insight poor.

The Canary Islands

On 17 January Bailey left Graylingwell for the first time in three years, for a weekend leave with his wife. Predictably, he became frightened and needed to return for a few days to his familiar refuge, but on the 29 January he was finally discharged 'cured' under Section 72 of the Mental Health Act and spent three weeks in Veta's flat in Worthing, which until then he had never seen. During this time, she drew him back to life by involving him in the next edition of *Short Practice*. Ever resourceful, Veta then arranged for them to fly three weeks later to Puerta de la Cruz in Tenerife, but this was not an ordinary holiday. They had never had any interest in going to some foreign country to 'relax', wander around buying souvenirs or lie on a beach. They had no interest in ancient history, painting or music. To Bailey, relaxation had been an opportunity to write, freed from the responsibilities of patient care. Veta chose Tenerife as the site for her husband's recuperation, but once there immediately engaged him in a debate on radio-isotopes, at that time a new concept in biology (though of course not in physics) and of no obvious immediate importance to surgeons. In spite of the assaults on his brain and his previous desperate illness, he was able to understand and comment on the new technology for the purposes of the next book, and write an account of it. While they were in the Canary Islands, an affectionate reconciliation between Hamilton and Veta took place and much of the bitterness of the past three years was healed.

Contact with the relaxed atmosphere of the Canary Islands undoubtedly paved the way for their later life in Southern Spain. There is no further record from Graylingwell, and we do not know whether or not the lithium was recommenced. In view of later experience, it would seem that to have discontinued the drug would have been most unwise, and indeed in May of that year, while Hamilton and Veta had come back to England and were spending a few weeks in Cornwall, she wrote to Dr Eddison saying that Hamilton had relapsed into depression with anorexia, insomnia and loss of concentration. Almost certainly, the lithium treatment was re-instituted, as from there on, although his mental health was perhaps not quite normal, the nightmare of the Graylingwell years was never repeated.

There was a somewhat pathetic attempt to return to active surgery. The terms of his contract with the Royal Northern, where he was now a member of the Emeritus Staff, entitled him to the use of five beds, and Bailey attempted to claim them. The Medical Defence Union, of which he was a life member, agreed the legal basis for the entitlement, but wisely refused any positive support for his case. The action petered out, to the benefit of the public, the profession and most certainly to Bailey himself. One suspects that he was in fact quite relieved at the outcome, and there can be no doubt that Veta would not have wished otherwise.

The Psychiatric Diagnosis

Bailey's diagnosis seems to have been that of mania, a condition which has a very strong hereditary tendency, so that in view of the family background it is not surprising that Bailey himself developed this type of problem in later life. In fact several diagnoses were made by the psychiatrists looking after him before and during his admission to Graylingwell. The first was that of a manic depressive psychosis, the second a mixed schizo-affective state and the third chronic paranoid schizophrenia. Dr Neil Joughin, Consultant Psychiatrist at Graylingwell, reviewed the notes for me and gave as his view that there was very little evidence to support a diagnosis of schizophrenia, apart from the fact that this diagnosis had already been applied to his sister May. Dr Joughin points out that the first rank symptoms described by Kurt Schnieder in the 1950s were none of them present in Bailey's case, and that the persecutory ideas which he had were relatively common also in mania. The spectacular response to Lithium again supports the diagnosis of what would now be termed 'Bipolar 1' disease. Dr Ian Daly in a leading article in *The Lancet* of April 1997 says:

> *The subjective experience of mania in its minor forms usually includes heightened feelings of well-being with increased alertness and drive, inflated self-esteem, and expansive sociability. In addition to a general elevation of mood, instability or lability is typical. Irritability may easily be evoked, and other mood states such as anxiety or sadness, fleetingly but intensely expressed, may become apparent. As mania deepens, over-activity and over-talkativeness become more obvious. Grandiose ideas and plans and grandiose delusions may develop.*

This seems to fit the case very well. Perhaps more interesting and remarkable is what happened after Bailey's discharge from Graylingwell, when the lithium treatment seems to have been discontinued completely. There was one minor relapse a few months later in Cornwall, but after this his mental state remained surprisingly stable, and the later years in Kent and in Spain seem to have been relatively tranquil. Difficult he certainly was, but the episodes of uncontrollability which made him unacceptable in society and precipitated his certification seemed never to have returned. Admittedly, the only evidence we have for this comes from Veta, and is second-hand, but the fact remains that the series of books and articles which flowed from his pen over this period could never have been accomplished by someone in the mental state of Bailey during his stay in Graylingwell.

Professor Guy Goodwin of Oxford University, an international authority who has made a special study of lithium and its effects, agrees that such an apparently complete recovery after what was a very short course of lithium is exceptional. Many patients who receive lithium early in their lives become worse if the treatment is withdrawn, However, in older patients this may not be the case, and up to 25% of cases do well.

Chapter 8

FINAL YEARS KENT AND SPAIN

Back to Work: Hull Place

On their return from The Canaries, Hamilton and Veta moved back to Worthing. Aunt Edith had left, but Veta's flat was still there, housing piles of records, transcripts and unopened correspondence. New books, new editions of old books, translations and requests for chapters in other peoples' books were lying around. They took up the old ways, working in adjoining rooms and comparing notes, but it soon became clear that this was not going to be possible and that they needed more space, if only to get away from each other during the day. Thanks to Veta's careful management, money was still coming in from the publishers, and following the sale of Denham they had no financial problems. Moreover, there were no dependents. Young Hamilton's death had seen to that.

In the early part of 1956 the Baileys moved to 4 Hull Place, Sholden, a few miles inland from Deal in Kent. Sholden was a small and, at that time, rather remote village surrounded by apple orchards and dairy farms, and Hull Place was an 18th-century manorial estate, whose out-buildings had been converted into dwellings. Number 4 is a comfortable red brick two-storey house set in an orchard. It provided an ideal retreat for Bailey, after the turmoil of the previous few years, where he could rest in privacy, gather his strength and take up the threads of the books. They built a small hut at the end of the garden, somewhat like the summerhouse at Totteridge, for Bailey to work in undisturbed. For her part, Veta no doubt hoped that a degree of isolation would afford her husband some respite from his mental turmoil, and give her a chance to put into practice the advice given by his psychiatrists. It is not known whether or not the lithium treatment was maintained, but those who knew Bailey at the time seem to think that it had been discontinued. If such was the case, it is surprising that there was no serious relapse of his illness. He was probably not stable, secure or happy, but he never again required admission to a mental hospital, and in view of his pathetic state during the first years in Graylingwell, the transformation was miraculous.

Editorial work on *Short Practice, Basic Surgery*, and *Pye*, continued. He resumed correspondence with his old house surgeon Alan Kark, now Professor of Surgery at the University of Natal in Durban. Kark had contributed chapters on snake bite and on heat stroke, and with his usual voracious reading of the literature Bailey came up with various bits of information which he sent back to Kark to enrich his contributions. For example, why did victims of snake bite not develop some form of immunity following repeated attacks? The answer seemed to be the prolonged intervals between bites, and the administration of antivenin, which inhibited the development of an immune response. Treatment in 1959 seemed still to be along the classical lines of a tourniquet, and incision and suction of the wound. Bailey comments that the occasional practices of treating a snake bite victim by transfusions from a person who had had similar bites in the past was 'obviously useless and to be condemned'. Similarly, he became interested in the use of concentrated solutions of urea in the management of head injuries. Head injuries cause death through swelling of the brain against the rigid confines of the skull, and if this is prevented, the vital centres which control breathing can be preserved. Urea reduces intracranial pressure by means of dehydration. It had been in use during brain operations for some time, but Bailey was one of the first to suggest its application in head injury, and the message duly appeared in Kark's chapter.

The years at Sholden were peaceful and productive. The couple established a daily routine, with Bailey working in the summerhouse through the morning, and having a walk and a nap in the afternoon. New editions of *Physical Signs* (translated into Chinese in 1956), *Short Practice, Emergency Surgery, Surgery for Nurses* and *Pye's Surgical Handicraft* all appeared during this period. Veta made friends with a photographer in Deal, a Mr Dunn, who enthusiastically joined in the work of editing the mass of clinical illustrations which arrived at Hull Place. Frequent trips to London were needed, to the Royal College of Surgeons, the Royal Society of Medicine (whose Librarian, Mr Bishop, collaborated with Bailey in many historical articles, and was co-author of *Notable Names in Medicine and Surgery*) the BMA and other repositories of knowledge. They usually went by train, but if the car was needed Veta was always the driver. No one at Sholden now remembers the Baileys, and it seems that they did not make many friends there. Hamilton had never enjoyed social small talk, and it is likely that there were times when he was depressed and uncommunicative.

Allan Clain, who had been first assistant at the Royal Northern, and was now a Consultant Surgeon at Dudley Road, and who had been of such support to Veta during Bailey's illness, was a frequent visitor to Hull Place, in his capacity as Editor of *Physical Signs* and of *Pye's Surgical Handicraft*. During Bailey's time in Graylingwell Veta had asked him to revise parts of the 12th edition of *Physical Signs*, but he soon found himself in sole responsibility, and ended up by editing the entire book. In fact, he later went on to revise and produce the 14th, 15th, 16th and 17th editions. Clain records how on one of his days at Sholden Bailey invited him to a local public house for a drink before lunch. During the walk across the marshes, the consumption of a half pint of beer and the walk back again, Bailey did not utter a single word.

To help him keep up to date and to gauge the effect of the books on the younger generation, he sounded them out before publication on the brighter students from his old medical school. Jack Hardcastle, now Professor of Surgery at Nottingham, was a student at The London in 1956, and he remembers writing commentaries on a proposed new edition, and receiving in return long and beautifully hand-written replies from Bailey. Sadly, no record of this correspondence remains. The books were by now so well known that each new edition was generally well received, but there were occasional setbacks. On 25 November 1959 Bailey wrote from Hull Place to his old friend Robert Cook of Bristol saying:

> *Dear Robert,*
>
> *Probably you have noticed the perfectly devastating review of basic surgery in this week's BMJ. It is written by John Bruce. I imagine this review will do the book a lot of harm, although I doubt whether it is having much say anyhow. I should think that Lewis' were very ill-advised to publish this; unless it was subsided they are likely to lose heavily on it. On the contrary, there are perfectly splendid reviews of* Short Practice - *not only in* Surgery, Gynecology and Obstetrics *but now in the* Annals of Surgery. *The review in* The Annals *is very long and entirely without adverse criticism. In fact, they recommend the book highly to U.S. readers...*

More follows about correspondence with a surgical registrar in Bombay, regarding surgical manifestations of guinea worm, and a curious condition known as ainhum, which results in gradual separation and loss of the fourth and fifth toes. Interestingly, the letter ends 'With all good wishes, Yours, Bill'. Very few people ever called Hamilton Bailey 'Bill' and certainly these did not include his wife. It was a name dating from his early career in Bristol, and reserved for very old friends such as Robert Cook.

Hawkinge

It is not quite certain why in early 1960 the Baileys gave up Hull Place, and moved to the Folkestone area. Perhaps it was simply because the lease came to an end, but there was a new annoyance. A small independent airline, the Silver City Line, had developed a flight path over the garden and the noise of the planes made it difficult for Bailey to dictate into his tape recorder (the Dictaphone had long since disappeared). But this was not the whole story. It seems that there were difficulties with the neighbours, which in view of Bailey's past medical history would not have been surprising. Additionally, Veta was becoming more and more limited by arthritis, and felt the need for somewhere smaller, and on one floor. For whatever reason, they moved to a bungalow called Long Meadow, in the village of Hawkinge, near Folkestone. Long Meadow included a swimming pool and a garden hut, convenient for writing, and correspondence with Kark and others continued from the new address. The letters to Kark (who had now left South Africa to take up the Chair of Surgery at Mount Sinai Hospital in New York) are revealing in their detail, and show a meticulous care for exactitude in illustration and in references. Thus on August 8:

> *Under separate cover I am sending proofs of your excellent chapter...I have made certain alterations to make it uniform with the rest of the book. In doing so I trust I have not altered your meaning in any way, but if so do not hesitate to correct.*

On October 5:

> *So at the moment I cannot say for certain, that what I am almost sure happened is that I put in the section you sent me in typescript on this subject, and I believe I altered it very slightly to indicate that an inhalation anaesthetic was essential if the patient was not deeply unconscious. I think I replied to you that I put this in italics.*

On October 20:

> *I am returning your transparency of gangrene following a snake bite. At your convenience, please let me know the type of snake that is likely to give a bite that leads to gangrene.*

On November 17:

> *Someone (I am almost certain that it was you) kindly sent me a transparency of a coloured boy with pyloric stenosis...on all colour prints I put a sticky label on the back saying who sent the original. In this particular instance the colour did not come out very well but I thought it an excellent photograph for the new edition of* Short Practice...*I am not sure whether this is your photograph or not, and that is what I am writing about.*

The signature to all these letters is firm, and where there are written annotations or footnotes the handwriting is neat and clear. These letters, all carefully typed by Veta, constantly refer to other correspondence, and one infers that dozens of letters must have poured out of Long Meadow every week. Veta's secretarial skills were in constant demand.

Fuengirola

It was at Hawkinge that they met Gillian Osborne and her husband who lived at Fuengirola in Southern Spain, but had come back for a short visit to England to see their family. The Osbornes explained the delights and advantages of life in the sun, and pressed Hamilton and Veta to visit them. The Baileys took up this offer and in early 1960 arrived in Fuengirola, where they put up at the Pensión Isabel owned by Maribel's sister, who later through Bailey's influence became a nurse at the Royal Northern. The Pensión, which still stands, later became a school for Swedish young ladies.

The Osbornes introduced Hamilton and Veta to their wide circle of friends, including a young architect, Ramon Morales. Morales sensed that they were interested in settling in the neighbourhood and offered to build them a house. They did not take long to decide. There was little now to keep them in England, money from the books was plentiful and in any case life in Spain was cheap, and they both liked the climate.

The result was the Baileys' first house in Spain, Las Golondrinas, built in 1960 on the northern edge of Fuengirola by Morales in association with a British architect called Carmichael (Figure 8.1).

The Baileys moved in and quickly established a social life. One of the sources of interest regarding the new arrivals was Hamilton's Rolls Royce, now

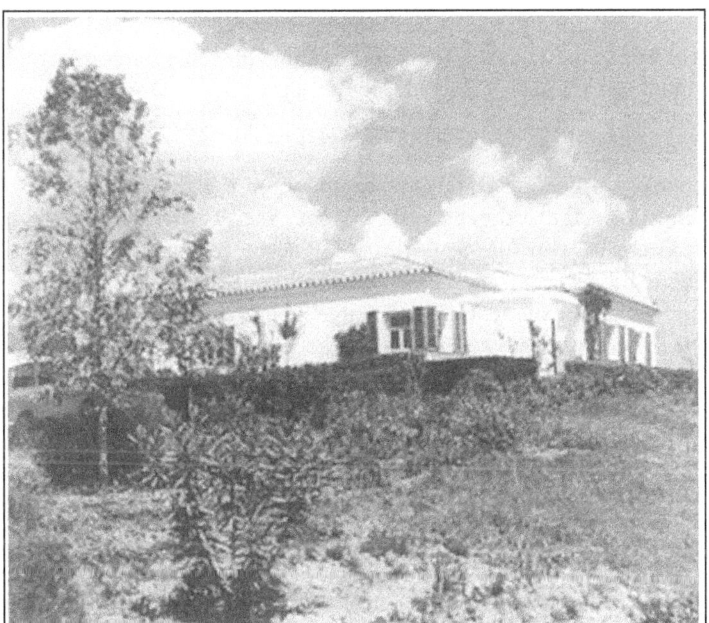

Figure 8.1: Las Golondrinas

rescued from storage, without a Dictaphone on the back seat, but nonetheless a striking and dramatic sight on the streets of a small Andalusian town, and a great conversation piece. Once again, Hamilton's reclusive nature was compensated by Veta who quickly made friends, among them San Bon Matsu, a Japanese-born artist married to a Spanish wife, and Don Manuel Verdugo, a much respected local General Practitioner who became their doctor. Don Manuel was an important figure in the community, whose patients erected a statue to him in the town square. Though now retired for many years, he remembers Bailey well, and his son has succeeded him in the practice. A young British architect, Aubrey David, was another friend, who described Bailey as 'a big, kind, gentle and considerate man, who never made the slightest effort to impress'. At one point the Davids asked him to see their small daughter, and were grateful for his skill and sympathy.

The Final Illness

The daily routine at Las Golondrinas was peaceful and orderly. The amenities were simple, but a warm climate and an undemanding pace of life made up for the lack of sophisticated pleasures. Veta entertained her friends, and Bailey continued to write and to receive colleagues and collaborators from abroad, and all seemed set for a quiet and undisturbed retirement. But the idyll was not to last. Early in January 1961, he began to experience attacks of abdominal pain and distension, to feel weak, to lose his appetite and then to lose weight. One morning he explained to Veta that he had had no bowel action for four days, something which was totally unusual for him. He felt well but, he said, 'if one of my patients came to me with this symptom, I would diagnose intestinal obstruction, which at my age is usually caused by cancer of the bowel'. Don Manuel was away at a medical conference in Madrid, and his assistant was called, who instructed the local District Nurse to administer an enema, which had no result. Because Bailey spoke no Spanish and Veta's command of the language was at an early stage, they decided that they should to Gibraltar to get their problem sorted out. Their approach was to the Senior Surgeon at the Colonial (later St Bernard's) Hospital in Gibraltar. This was D. J. Toomey (Figure 8.2) a man of very considerable stature and experience. For a surgeon in a small, closed community of 25 000 people to preserve confidence and keep a sound reputation is exceedingly difficult, as successes tend to be forgotten and the slightest mistake is invariably magnified and remembered. In spite of this, Toomey had maintained a position of great respect in the community for 20 years, and the later award of an OBE acknowledged his achievement.

Bailey telephoned Toomey and spoke to his wife, Edna. His words were: 'to think I have written about this so often and yet now feel I have to ask someone else about it - I have noticed increasing constipation'. Toomey insisted that they come immediately to Gibraltar. He arranged Bailey's admission to St Bernard's, while Veta put up at a small pension, the Haven Court, which was next to the

Garrison Library. Each day she walked up the steep narrow streets of Gibraltar to the hospital, although advised by Toomey to stay at the Rock Hotel (which she could easily have afforded) and visit by taxi.

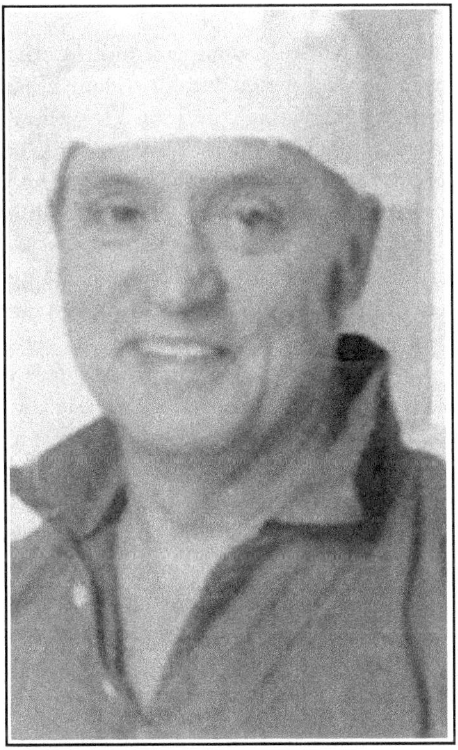

Figure 8.2: D. J. Toomey in 1961

Bailey was still a big strong man, and a physical examination did not show any particular sign of ill health. However the history and symptoms indicated a problem in the colon, and Toomey arranged for a barium enema to be carried out in the first instance, later to be followed by a barium meal, if the result was negative. Bailey however was adamant that these tests should be done in the reverse order, and Toomey acquiesced. The barium meal showed a narrowed area about three inches long in the lower part of the colon, at the point where it joins the rectum. The upper part of the colon was not dilated, and the appearances were typical of the very common condition known as diverticular disease, in which there is infection of small outpouchings of the bowel lining. Toomey came to the X-ray department and told Bailey that he should now have a barium enema, to which he replied 'we don't need to do that when I can see clearly that it is just an area of diverticulosis. Anyway, I have to get back to Spain and I am working on my latest revision of *Pye's Surgical Handicraft*. He insisted on leaving. Possibly Veta's uncomfortable lodgings at Haven Court, about which she was always complaining, had some part in that decision. Toomey was hesitant to let him go, but Bailey was as usual dominating and insistent. 'If you have any further trouble please ring me and I will come up to Fuengirola and collect you' was Toomey's departing remark. This was no problem as at that time the Spanish frontier was open and Toomey drove a powerful Jaguar.

When Bailey arrived back in Fuengirola it was clear that the problem was unresolved. His constipation continued and his abdomen began to distend. Dr Verdugo was sent for, and unhesitatingly diagnosed large bowel obstruction. He called in Dr Lopez, one of the prominent younger surgeons in Malaga, who agreed with the diagnosis and admitted Bailey urgently to his private clinic. The diagnosis of acute obstruction of the large bowel was now absolutely clear, as was the need for an immediate operation. However this was no ordinary patient, and it was not easy to take quick decisions. There were prolonged discussions. At times, Bailey would become submissive and obedient, and put himself unreservedly in the hands of his surgeon. On other occasions he would quite unpredictably attempt to take charge, and tell the doctors what to do. Eventually, after five days delay, he agreed to the operation, but refused to have any sort of colostomy. Dr Lopez was then faced with the problem of operating on an elderly sick man with an obstructed, distended and septic colon. He would no doubt have preferred to carry out a preliminary artificial opening, so as to decompress the bowel and allow it to be joined up later when circumstances would have been so much more favourable, but his patient would not agree. Bailey's decision to countermand this was ironic in view of his well known preference for 'staged' approaches to surgery, and indeed to much of his writing. In the event, Lopez operated and found a tumour at the exact point in the rectosigmoid which the barium meal had indicated. He diagnosed cancer and in obedience to his patient's instructions, he resected the tumour, joined up the colon and closed the abdomen.

The result could have been foretold from any of Bailey's books, and is all too familiar to surgeons who work on the colon. The anastomosis leaked, peritonitis and a faecal fistula developed, he became febrile, toxic and shocked, and several more drastic operations were carried out in a desperate attempt to reverse what soon became a clearly irretrievable situation. It must be remembered that at that time the understanding of fluid balance and maintenance of surgical metabolism was at a fairly primitive stage, and furthermore that broad-spectrum antibiotics were not universally available.

During all of this Bailey was entirely aware of what was happening, and must have appreciated his desperate plight. Nonetheless, his main preoccupation, even to the end, seemed to be the production of the latest textbook, and the new editions of *Pye's Surgical Handicraft* and the *Short Practice of Surgery*, were still underway. We have no record of what Veta went through during these final agonising days.

Toomey came up from Gibraltar. He was appalled at what had happened. It appeared that Bailey had been told that he had a volvulus of the colon (a volvulus is a simple mechanical twist, easily corrected by surgery). Toomey knew well that this was not the case, as he had the X-ray with him, which he gave to Veta (a decision he later regretted). Veta explained that Hamilton must not be unduly disturbed or worried, because of his psychiatric problems, and the trauma occasioned by young Hamilton's death. Toomey goes on to say:

> *It was horrible to see this famous man alone in a darkened room with no one to speak English with. I returned to tell Edna that I thought he was going to die, and when we returned on the Friday I knew he was. He told me he had had seven operations since I had seen him last. It was pathetic. I came out of the Clinic to find Edna. I said 'he is finished'. I then had a stroke of luck to meet in the street, while we were talking, the Spanish Psychiatric Consultant who visited Gibraltar. He telephoned the surgeon whom he knew well and arranged for me to see him later. He said he had found HB had an annular carcinoma. I knew this to be untrue, ...know that even at operation one can feel an area of diverticular disease it can be difficult to state categorically it was not a carcinoma. However, the deed was done. I said 'should he not have blood ?' 'We do not believe in giving blood in Spain !' His electrolytes were being balanced by giving him oral Coca Cola (23 bottles a day). He said he could send HB to any hospital in London, but I realised that his next step was the cemetery - and so it was!*

Hamilton Bailey died in Málaga on 26 March 1961.

Toomey's final comment was 'a proximal transverse colostomy would have saved HB's life and he could have had the greatest surgeon of his choice to carry out the elective procedure'. This was certainly true, and to some extent Bailey contributed to his own demise. What a tragic end to the life of a great surgeon. Having recovered from a massive mental illness, complicated by chemical and electrical assaults on his brain, he finally makes his own diagnosis, but falters at the last stage in taking clinical charge of his own body. Instinctively, he knew that he had lower bowel obstruction, and that a barium meal was not the appropriate examination. However, perhaps because of unwillingness to accept the truth, perhaps because of his obsessive preoccupation with his writing, he both bullies his colleagues and colludes with them. When the barium meal is followed down to the colon and discloses an apparently benign stricture, he accepts the diagnosis, and refuses the barium enema which in his heart of hearts he knows is the next required step. Two days later this fatal mistake catches up with him. We cannot blame Toomey, a meticulous and conscientious surgeon, somewhat in awe of his preceptor. Nor indeed can we criticise Dr Lopez, forced against his better judgement by this world famous colleague to carry out an operation which he would find hard to justify in print or at a medical meeting. As complications developed, Bailey discusses each one with his surgeon, and acquiesces in each new fruitless intervention. He knew he was going to die and at some point must have said 'well - enough is enough, let us leave things alone'. We will never know the true diagnosis, which in any case is by now a matter of small importance. Even if the part of the colon which was removed was ever sent to a pathology laboratory, the report is not available. But cancer is by far the most frequent cause of colonic obstruction of the type which affected Bailey, and Dr Lopez' diagnosis was almost certainly correct.

The British Cemetery at Málaga

Up until 1830, all infidels dying in Málaga had been buried on the beach, with their feet pointing out to sea. Infidels historically included Moslems and Jews, and there had been very little contact with Protestants until that time. The British Consul, William Mark, was devoted to Málaga, which he described as a second paradise, and encouraged his compatriots to settle there, and in order to assure them of a decent interment should the need arise, succeeded in negotiating the establishment of a British cemetery. The inscription above the door reads:

> *CEMETERIO INGLES*
> ***Establecido por Real Orden de Su Majestad Católica de 11 Abril de 1830, en confirmación á la cesión hecha a Don Guillermo Mark, Consul de su Majestad Británica para la Region de Granada por el General Don Jose Manso, Gobernador de Málaga etc etc etc.***

The portal is surmounted by a cross, which rather surprised the locals at the time, as they had assumed that the Protestants were a Jewish sect. Mark had to wait two years before his first corpse arrived, but after that the cemetery filled up with deceased invalids and drowned sailors. The first graves were small and primitive but as the British community grew and prospered more sumptuous tombs appeared, and a beautiful garden developed around them. The place was further embellished by Mark's son, and became a tourist attraction. Following his visit Hans Christian Andersen wrote 'I can well understand how a splenetic Englishman might take his own life in order to be buried in this place'. Bailey's tomb is in a quiet shady corner of the cemetery, surrounded by the graves of wine shippers and retired naval officers. Veta lies there too, but did not wish to have her name recorded on the headstone.

As news of the death emerged, letters of condolence poured in to Las Golondrinas from all over the world. A memorial plaque to Bailey was put up in the Parque San Antonio Hospital in Málaga, and his photograph hangs in the International College of Surgeons in Chicago. Obituaries appeared in *The Lancet*, *British Medical Journal* and *British Journal of Surgery*. A bookcase of memorabilia was set up at the Royal Northern Hospital, and when the new operating theatres were opened there many years later in 1970, they were named after him, together with McNeill Love (Figure 8.3).

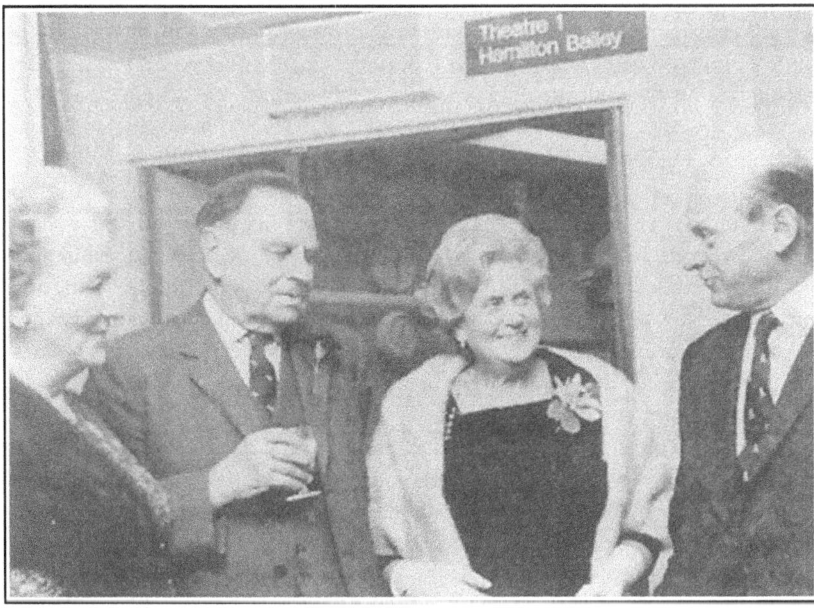

Figure 8.3: Opening of the St David's Wing Operating Suite, 1968

Mijas

Hamilton had always been the mainspring of Veta's life, but she at the same time had fuelled his inspiration and been his principal support. Having lost her only son many years ago and now her husband, and living in a foreign country whose language she did not speak, it would have been easy for her to return to Britain, perhaps look for a new companion, or decline into genteel widowhood in Bournemouth or Cheltenham. The deprivation was colossal, but so also were the challenges, the new freedoms and opportunities, and with her husband's death a burden had been lifted. Veta decided to re-create a life for herself in her new found country. The books were selling well and she was not short of money.

She and Hamilton had chosen to build their house in Fuengirola, but the town was beginning to expand around them, and they had often thought of moving up into the hills a few miles outside, to Mijas. Mijas is a long white village extending along the slope of the Sierra Nueva. When the Baileys first went there in 1961 it was a comparatively primitive place, reached only by a narrow twisting mountain road up from Fuengirola. Although poor and isolated, Mijas was a place of great beauty and had already attained some international fame because of an extraordinary story dating from the Civil War. When the Spanish Republic was declared in 1931, the village barber, Manuel Cortes, a lifelong socialist, had been elected deputy Mayor by a large majority. Although an atheist who welcomed the reforming aspects of Republican policy and particularly relaxation of the divorce laws and the introduction of civil marriage, he was always firmly democratic, and was certainly not the dangerous Bolshevík depicted in the right wing press. Cortes became Mayor just at the outbreak of the Civil War, and when the insurgent forces under Franco overran his village, went into hiding in the mountains. He later secretly returned to a minute upstairs room in his own house in Mijas, concealed and cared for by his family and neighbours. During the whole of the Second World War and the ensuing dictatorship, in danger of his life, Cortes remained in hiding. Only on the death of Franco and the re-establishment of democracy in 1968 did he emerge, having spent 33 years in his one small room. Coming out of his place of concealment he was dumbfounded by the transformation that had occurred not only in his own pueblo, which was by now overrun with tourists, but also by the transformation of Fuengirola from a simple fishing village into an international resort, with massive concrete hotels and busloads of foreigners.

Veta had always delighted in Mijas, and was now determined to live there. Mijas was virtually two villages, the east being the traditional Spanish community and the west the nucleus of a new expatriate suburb. The halves of the village did not always associate. At that time there were very few British expatriates, according to her friend Charles Beamish as few as eight or ten. Veta discovered a small site on the upper slopes of the west village and in association with the British architect Aubrey David, who had been a close friend of the Baileys when they lived in Fuengirola, she built Los Arcos. At that time the house stood almost alone on the edge of the village, with a magnificent view down to the Mediterranean. Los Arcos is still there, although the view has been interrupted by surrounding buildings. It is compact, but generously planned, with a beautiful pergola and balcony, and bourgainvillea and vines climbing up the white walls. Veta installed herself, looked after by her gardener Ernesto and his wife Lázara, and although she spoke no Spanish became quickly respected and liked by the local population because of her transparently generous character. Very soon she began to exert her influence on the small but expanding British expatriate community and became known as outgoing, generous, charitable, and always available to new arrivals. She took trouble to organise their social lives, introduced them to like-minded people, and helped to guide them through the local bureaucracy while they were becoming established, and soon became acknowledged as their social leader. A particular friend was Charles Beamish, an accountant who had spent many years in South America and had retired to Mijas in 1966. Typically, as soon as Veta met him through friends, she invited him to a party. There were few English people in Mijas at that time and Beamish was not particularly anxious to become part of the expatriate clan. Rather reluctantly he came to her party but such was her charm that from that moment onwards they saw much of each other and became close friends. Over the next few years Beamish helped her with her financial affairs and with those of the Bailey foundation, with her social life and engagements, letters and typing. Eventually they had a joint bank account: he describes Veta as a wonderful person, generous, helpful, outgoing and immensely sociable.

Some members of the English community had surgical backgrounds and had known Hamilton. These included Rainsford Mowlem the plastic surgeon from The Middlesex, and the daughter of Professor d'Abreu from Birmingham, who later married the writer Roald Dahl. The Irish Surgeon O'Malley was a close neighbour. She kept in touch with her friends from Fuengirola including Gill Osborne, her husband and her daughter Suzanne, the Verdugo medical family, and San Bon Matsu, who lived with his wife and daughter in the Edificio Bolero in downtown Fuengirola. He had known Veta since the very early days of her arrival in the Pensión Isabel, though he never knew Hamilton well. A friend of the Verdugo family and a man of wide acquaintance in the town, he was very useful to Veta in her social aspirations and, was extremely kind and valuable to her in the hard times to come.

Veta's social life in Mijas flourished and expanded. She entertained widely, and her vitality, charm and generosity became legendary (Figure 8.4). Everybody in Mijas remembers her. Her maid Lázara and gardener Ernesto remained eight years with Veta in Mijas and when she returned to Fuengirola came back to serve her for another eight years. They describe her as an exacting but generous employer. She became closely associated with Aubrey David and his family and was godmother to the David children. The children regarded her as an honorary aunt, and always referred to her as Auntie Veta, to the extent that some of the Mijas people thought that her name was 'Antiveta'. There were parties at her house at which her famous Dalmatian Jonathan was a frequent participant.

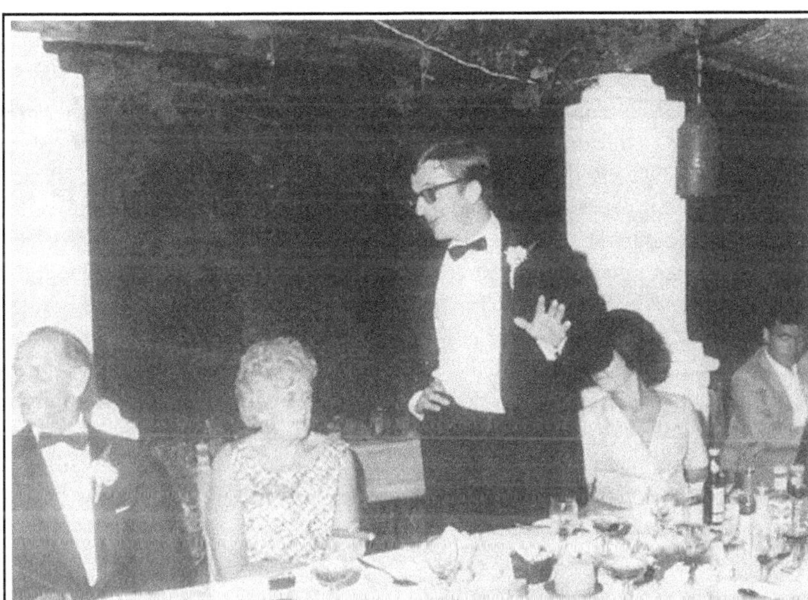

Figure 8.4: Veta socialising

During all these busy years in Mijas Veta never ceased to work on the books and to preserve her husband's memory through his writings. One of her deepest regrets was to discover, among his papers, plans for a new book on parotid surgery, with chapter headings, text and illustrations, which was however not in publishable form. John Lumley, Allan Clain, Alan Kark, Anthony Raines with his two daughters and many others were regular visitors to Los Arcos, where they enjoyed Veta's hospitality, and discussed new avenues for publication and the distribution of the royalties. Not all of these discussions were easy and straightforward. For instance there was a disagreement with Allan Clain regarding the 14th editon of *Physical Signs*, which was eventually happily resolved, and Clain went on to edit the 15th, 16th and 17th editions. The Hamilton Bailey Trust was set up by Veta in conjunction with the accountant Brian Worth, who was one of Hamilton's executors. The Trust continues to this day, and distributes charitable money all over the world. Its precise activities are discussed in detail in the epilogue.

Another visitor at Los Arcos was Margaret Bailey's sister Edith, the Aunt Edith who had been so good to Hamilton in the difficult days in Worthing before his admission to Graylingwell. She was visited by Charles Beamish at her home in Essex, shortly before she died at the age of 92. Although pleased and proud to talk about her husband, Veta never referred to his mental illness or other darker moments of his life. No one that I met in Mijas remembers hearing about the tragedy of young Hamilton.

Life continued in Los Arcos in this way until 1978, when for reasons which are not altogether clear, Veta decided that a move was necessary. Aubrey David was constructing an 'urbanisation' in Estepona, a few miles down the coast, and interested Veta in the project. The plan was for Veta to buy two villas, one of which she was to live in and the other was to be rented. Somehow or other, this plan never came to fruition. The rights and wrongs of the matter are difficult to determine, and clearly there is still a major difference of opinion between Veta's friends in Fuengirola and the David family. It seemed unnecessarily intrusive for Hamilton's biographer to risk opening old wounds in an attempt to unravel this situation, which occurred several years after his death. Whatever happened, the upshot was that Veta returned to Fuengirola and took an apartment in the Edificio Bolero, immediately above the one occupied by San Bon Matsu. The Matsu family were unswervingly kind and supportive to Veta during subsequent years of her life during which she developed cataracts and became almost immobilised with arthritis. She was nonetheless maintained in her popularity in the region and one of the last photographs of her shows her at the celebration of the unveiling of the bust to Dr Verdugo in Fuengirola, in her wheelchair and flanked by her friends and supporters (Figure 8.5).

Veta died on the 4 February 1990, and her ashes were taken by Charles Beamish to lie in Hamilton's tomb in the English cemetery in Málaga. At her request, her name was not added to his on the headstone of the grave.

There is a mysterious episode in the Baileys' life, which has defied investigation. It seems that they might have adopted one, or even two, daughters. Such a wish would have been easy to understand, given what had happened to them, though one would question whether this gravely troubled couple were really in a position to care for a small girl. During their time in Kent there were rumours

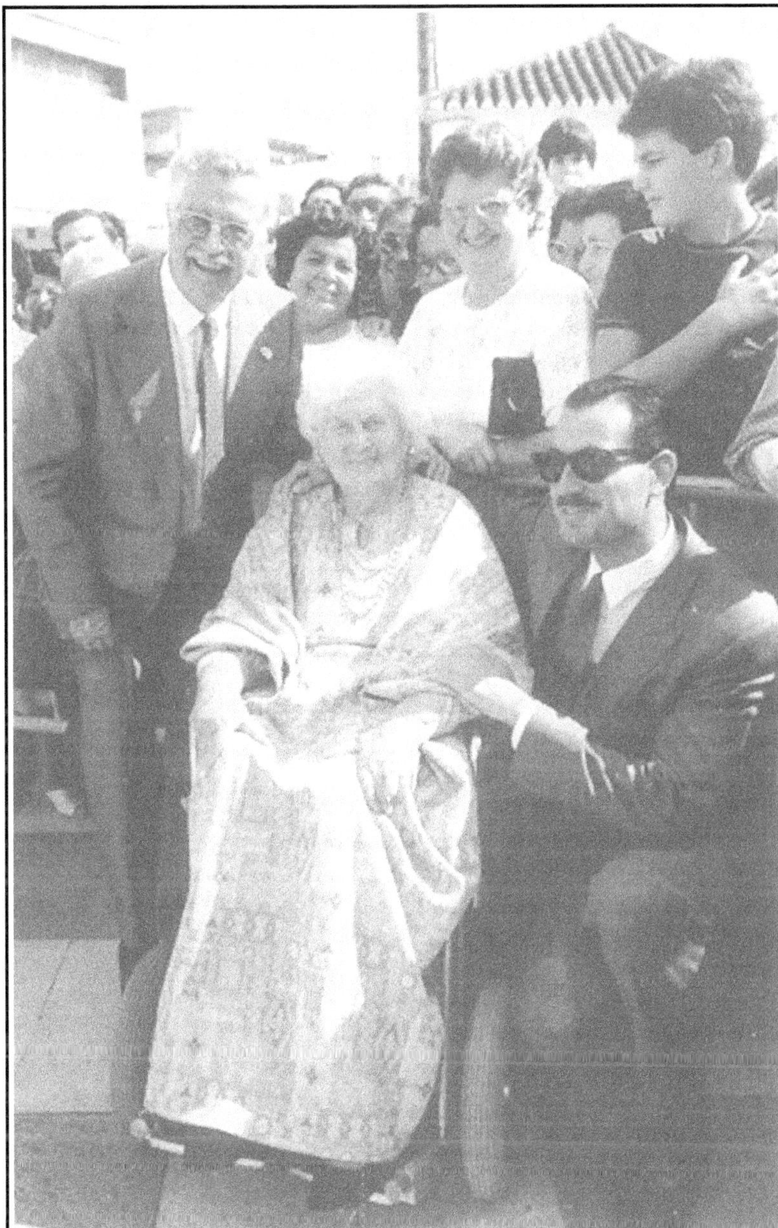

Figure 8.5. Veta with Don Manuel Verdugo and Dr Juan Verdugo, at the unveiling of Don Manuel's bust in Fuengirola, a few weeks before she died

of a young Australian who had joined them in the house, but had later been sent back to her parents. It seems very unlikely that Veta would have entered into a contractual adoptive relationship, and what is much more probable is that they employed some sort of an 'au pair', who subsequently returned home. Even more mysterious is the rumour that after Hamilton's death Veta travelled to Bombay and came back with an adopted Indian girl. Charles Beamish was close to Veta during the whole of her life in Mijas and has no recollection of the event, and the only source of information is from Zina Fitzgerald, who remembers meeting an Indian girl at Los Arcos on two occasions. She gained the impression that this was an adopted daughter, but no one else in Mijas has confirmed her view.

The Trusts

When the Baileys first arrived in Spain, in spite of Hamilton's apparent wellbeing in the warm Mediterranean climate, both of them were concerned about his future physical and mental health, so that they decided to set up a Trust and a Company to make certain that, whatever happened, Veta would be continue to receive an income, and at the same time would be able to carry on Hamilton's work. All of the books were selling well and royalties were steadily coming in. The problem was not one of income, but rather of how to deal with the money in the most prudent way.

The Trust, which still exists, was called the Hamilton Bailey Medical Libraries. Its prime purpose is to donate books to medical schools in developing countries. The originally trustees were Veta, Alan Clain, John Hawkins (solicitor to Veta and also incidentally to the Medical Defence Union) and Brian Worth. Worth, who was a recently qualified accountant, took on the Bailey Trust funds as his first major job. He never met Hamilton, but was later to prove a true and valuable friend to Veta.

Some 200 medical schools throughout the world were identified and approached. Those that responded favourably and have benefited from the Trust include Mona University at Kingston, Jamaica, the Christian Medical College of South India at Vellor, Seth College in Bombay, The Khyber Medical College at Peshawar, and the Medical School of Papua New Guinea. The work continues to this day. Around 1986, the Trust approached the Royal College of Surgeons with the suggestion that they take over its funds and responsibilities. The response of the College was somewhat equivocal and the Trust was invited to support the STEP (Surgical Trainees Educational Programme) course. Negotiations continue.

Quite apart from the Trust, Veta and Brian Worth set up a Company (HB Medical Works Ltd) which administers the proceeds from Hamilton Bailey's books and assured Veta of an income during her lifetime. The company owned some of the copyrights, for example, *Short Practice of Surgery*, which was held for the lifetime of Hamilton and Veta, and has now reverted to the publishers, Chapman & Hall. The company has a present a capital of some £500 000, derived from royalties and investment profits. Four books continue in publication, including *Pye's Surgical Handicraft*, *Emergency Surgery*, *Physical Signs* and the *Short Practice of Surgery*. In an informal way, the company helps to fund young British surgeons who wish to travel abroad. This arrangement is conducted in association with the International College of Surgeons.

About 18 months before she died, Veta created a second Trust, The Veta Bailey Charitable Trust, the terms of which are quite loose, and are not confined to medical charities. Under the terms of Veta's will the company was wound up, half of its assets going to the Medical Libraries Trust, whose good work continues, the other half remaining with the charity, which is administered by Brian Worth, and by Dr Elizabeth MacClatchy of Belfast. In 1994 the Trust contributed £65 000 to medical training in the third world.

EPILOGUE

Why do young men and women want to become doctors? It would be comfortable to imagine that they are driven by a wish to alleviate human suffering, to reveal the origins of disease and to advance the cause of health. While this may be true of a minority, it does not match the experience of those who teach 19 year old entrants to medical training, who see a quite different pattern of motivation in their students. The students are selected on purely educational grounds, that is the "levels" which they have obtained in their school examinations. Compassion is not in the syllabus, which is probably just as well. A profession recruited from immature idealists would not save many lives. In fact, most young medical students seem to be driven by a desire for a stable career and a respected place in society, peer group pressure from schoolfriends who are doing the same thing, family traditions and family ambitions. Others come into the profession because of an enquiring mind and an interest in science, but in fact the only students in whom altruism is conspicuous are those mature entrants who, often at considerable sacrifice, opt for medicine in their twenties or thirties, or even later, as a second career.

Beyond that, what makes a young doctor become a surgeon? Ideally it should be a discovery of inherited manual skills which can be put to good use in helping the sick. Most people would expect that manual dexterity would be a surgeon's most important criterion for advancement. Most people would prefer to be operated on by an unsympathetic master craftsman rather than face mutilation or loss of life at the hands of a kind and charming blunderer. Most people would assume that young surgeons are carefully assessed with regard to their handling of instruments and tissues, and are selected and promoted because of their skill in the operating theatre. Each of these notions is wrong. Medical trainees choose a surgical career for all sorts of reasons, the glamour and prestige of the craft being one of the most important, and are in their turn then chosen for a range of abilities, only one of which is that of manual skill. Success in the profession is measured by the capacity to diagnose illness, teach students and postgraduates, organise and manage a department, carry out and publish research, befriend colleagues and officials, avoid litigation, earn money for and add to the prestige of the parent institution. Paradoxically, although it is the surgeons who operate the selection procedure, they often see little of each others' work in the theatre. It is the anaesthetists who really know who the good ones are.

Hamilton Bailey chose surgery because it appealed to his instincts for direct, simple action rather than analysis. He was not especially dexterous, and those who came to watch him operate, drawn by his fame as a teacher and writer, were often disappointed. His anaesthetists, with the possible exception of Donald Blatchley who was a special case, did not esteem him highly.

Unfairly, but perhaps as no surprise, the image of the surgeon has changed from hero to villain. The Dr Kildare of the 1960s, tireless, idealistic, compassionate and always right, has been replaced in television series and tabloid newspapers by the elderly arrogant self seeker, out of touch with his patients and failing in his personal life, whose incompetence is shored up by a professional conspiracy on the part of his colleagues. Books with titles such as "The Romance of Surgery" and "The Century of the Surgeon", so popular in the 1970s, could never be published today. Both extremes are of course equally misleading: surgeons are no better or worse than anyone else, but their uniquely responsible and conspicuous place in society exposes them to the sort of pressure which is not experienced by other health professionals.

The notorious "Medical Duckshoot Story" has been told so many times after so many dinners that a speaker who embarks on it is now greeted with groans of disapproval, but bears repetition here. The story goes as follows. A physician, a psychiatrist, a surgeon and a pathologist went out one morning to shoot ducks. As they stood waiting, a bird came over. The physician said "Maybe that is a duck. But there again, maybe it is not. What test, investigation or analysis can I carry out to settle the matter? Should it be a computerised scan, a double isotope study or a simple megakaryocyte count?" By that time the bird had flown away. The psychiatrist's turn was next. As the bird came into sight the psychiatrist mused "Maybe that is a duck. But what makes me think that? Could it be some repressed anxiety or some event in my early childhood which is influencing me? Am I perhaps ducking the truth? Perhaps my mother did not love me enough?" By the time that he had finished these reflections the bird had vanished. Another one appeared. The surgeon shot it down, turned to the pathologist and asked "What was that?"

Naturally, pathologists love to tell this tale which makes a simple but not altogether unfair point. Bailey was the archetypal man of action rather than of thought, and contemplation of a problem bored him. This swiftness of purpose impressed his pupils and earned him the approbation of the local doctors, and who is to say that they were wrong, given the circumstances of the time?

Hamilton Bailey did not become a surgeon through idealism or religious conviction but rather because given his family background, it was the obvious thing to do. Once in medical school, he discovered in himself an intense curiosity in the natural world and a range of intellectual talents which he was delighted to exploit. Seeing him in 1925, an energetic young registrar with an FRCS and a good war record, one would have predicted a smooth ascent up the surgical career ladder, ending in the prestigious appointment at a London teaching hospital which he had always desperately wanted. But things did not work out in this way.

The crucial position of the London teaching hospitals deserves some explanation. Medicine is now taught where it is mainly practised, that is to say in GP surgeries and in district hospitals. The distinction between teaching institutions and the others has largely disappeared, as all hospitals receive students. Things were very different in the first half of the century, and indeed at the inception of the National Health Service in 1948 a clear distinction was made between an elite group of teaching hospitals, which retained their Boards of Governors and their accumulated funds, and had direct access to the Department of Health, and those hospitals which were managed by a local health authority. In London, the twelve great hospitals had developed their own medical schools which in many cases had antedated the foundation of the University, and their consultants had a unique status and power which was equivalent to, and in some respects greater than, that of the Professors, partly because their private earnings made them much richer. The schools were linked to, but independent of, the University and were able to dictate the ways in which students and specialists were trained. The situation was in total contrast to that on the continent of Europe, where both undergraduate and postgraduate training has always been in the hands of the Universities, and the Professor is the undisputed chief. In this country, it was the teaching hospitals which recruited undergraduate medical students, set their examinations and assessed them. Their consultant staff provided the governing bodies of the Royal Colleges of Physicians and Surgeons, which had for centuries retained statutory authority to grant diplomas and licences to practice that were recognised by government. The teaching hospitals, moreover, held a monopoly of research, through their university links and inherited wealth and, since an intending specialist needed to train at one of them, they were able to cream off the most able and energetic graduates, which in turn fuelled their power and prestige. For an ambitious young surgeon such as Bailey, to secure a consultant appointment at one of these hospitals was a prime objective, and his unsuccessful attempts at Bristol and Birmingham and eventually, most importantly, at his own training school, The London, led to a corroding sense of bitterness and resentment, almost amounting to persecution, which must have contributed to the tragic events of the 1960s. Was Veta in part responsible? Alan Clain, who knew them both well, comments: "there is no doubt that [Veta] supplied much of Bailey's drive and whereas he might have ended up happily as a surgeon at a provincial hospital in the course of time, she encouraged him in the endeavours which led to his failures to get on to the consultant staff of a teaching hospital successively at the London, Liverpool, Birmingham and Bristol. I also know that in 1947 he applied for the Chair of Surgery in Cape Town, which went to a local nonentity".

Beyond any doubt, the reasons which lay behind Bailey's failure to gain acceptance by colleagues in his own country and by the British medical establishment, lay in the complex and difficult character of the man.

In the first place there was the background of mental illness. We do not know the diagnosis (in present-day terms) of his mother's condition, nor that of his sister May, though she would almost certainly nowadays be labelled as schizophrenic. Psychiatric labels change with time, but the one which seems to have been most often applied to Bailey in the 1950s most accurately is that of mania, a condition which is still defined and recognised as a variant of bipolar disease. Quite apart from the legacy of mental illness, Bailey inherited a personality which made it difficult for him to be liked by his fellow creatures. Although he had a penetrating intellect and a tremendous capacity for absorbing knowledge, he lacked imagination, and seems not to have the least trace of a sense of humour. Perhaps imagination and humour were tender plants, which were suppressed by the harsh treatment he received in early life. His father was busy, remote and preoccupied, and his mother's tempestuous unreliability is a matter of record. What did he make of his little sister's being concealed from the public as someone embarrassing and shameful, and being sent away to an asylum at such an early age? It was always obvious to him that he might one day himself "go mad" as he would have put it and this comes out clearly in the letters written from Graylingwell. In later life, he had an enormous circle of acquaintanceships and colleagues to whom he wrote warmly professional letters, but he had very few real friends. His relationship with McNeill Love, with whom he had shared years of frustration and adversity, and with whom he collaborated so closely when the tide of publications began to flow, was cold and distant. Critics have accused him of having taken little affectionate interest in young Hamilton, and his feelings following the catastrophe of July 1943 seem at first sight to have been more those of remorse and guilt rather than of grief at the loss of a loved young companion. He had always sensed the danger of madness, and had developed a system of self protection, but the death of his son was too much to bear, and the shell was cracked open.

Finally, what of Veta? Scattered throughout the record there are many scraps of evidence indicating devotion and tenderness from her to him, but there is absolutely nothing coming from the other side. Perhaps Veta destroyed his letters. It would be wrong to pass judgement, but a lack of reciprocated tenderness was entirely consistent with the character that emerges from the rest of the story. Veta certainly inspired and disciplined Bailey's activities, but the picture of the over-ambitious wife who insensitively drove her husband to develop expectations which he could never fulfil is both simplistic, and very unfair. Not only was she a more sympathetic person than Hamilton, but also her talents were broadly based, and her capacity to like and to be liked by other people enabled her to take much fuller advantage of the social opportunities arising from his work than he himself would ever have achieved, and to develop a mature and satisfying old age. Would this have been possible if he had survived?

To his patients, Bailey was charitable and honourable, but not kind or understanding. They in turn respected him and trusted his ability, but did not like him He worked hard to support the interests and careers of his junior colleagues, in the sense of writing letters and testimonials, but was so impatient with incompetent behaviour that he did not earn their affection, trust or loyalty. On the other hand, there is nowhere the least trace of malice, intrigue or vindictiveness. Although he might wound the feelings of a young doctor or nurse by his impatience with anyone who failed to meet his high standards or carry out his instructions to the letter, this was the result of insensitivity rather than any desire to wound. He contributed generously to charities and although the books brought in much wealth, he had no interest in accumulating money, except to the extent that a reasonable income would enable him to pursue his life's work in writing and teaching.

What in fact were Bailey's contributions to medicine? He was, essentially, a scientist. This may seem a strange claim to make in respect of someone who never entered a laboratory since his student days, and never conducted an experiment. Science, however, is as much advanced by observation as by experiment, and Bailey was a supreme observer. He was obsessed by the function and more particularly the structure of the human body, and was a brilliant applied anatomist. His knowledge of the interior of the body enabled him to use his eyes and hands in solving a clinical problem in a way which was unique and unrivalled, and he was able to translate those skills into books which went all over the world, and are still currently in print, with new editions planned. Although their content and authorship have totally changed, and it is unlikely that the 1996 edition of *Bailey and Love* contains many words written by either of them, the impact of these two names is as potent as ever.

Bailey's one anatomical discovery was in fact erroneous. This concerned the anatomy of the parotid gland, which he described as being rather like a "cottage loaf" with the branches of the facial nerve running between the two hemispheres. This false concept was the basis of his operation for removal of tumours of the gland, an operation which succeeded, for quite the wrong reasons. His other scientific contributions involve the use of blood transfusion, the anatomy and surgery of branchial cysts, and the organisation of an out-patient urology clinic. One of his most influential books was *The Surgery of Modern Warfare*, in which he reiterated the message of delayed primary suture (see Chapter 4). Additionally, he was one of the first surgeons to devise an organised drill to deal with cardiac arrest. This emergency does not permit of hesitation or reflection and often occurs when there are no skilled staff around - what is required is a procedure which can be put into practice swiftly and automatically, regardless of who is carrying it out, and Bailey very easily appreciated the need which often arises to act on instinct rather than evidence. That these concepts were the result of practical experience informed by a distillation of papers from the international literature does not detract from their originality or value.

As in a Greek tragedy the element of hubris caught up with this turbulent and defiant man. His early death was quite unnecessary. Although he undoubtedly had a cancer of the colon, there is nothing to suggest that the tumour had spread, and he did not die of cancer as such, but rather from an obstruction of the bowel. The extent to which surgeons can cure cancer is problematic, but no one can deny their ability to deal with obstructed tubes, as Bailey had done on many occasions. It was his surgical knowledge and eminence which disturbed the judgement of the doctors treating him, both in Gibraltar and Spain. Had he understated his identity, or submissively put himself in the hands of the clinicians, the outcome would probably have been quite different. His blocked colon would have been relieved by a colostomy, following which the cancer would have been assessed and probably quite easily removed. This would not have guaranteed survival, but would at least would have given him a better chance. On the other hand, had he chosen to pull rank, and insist that as the foremost world authority on emergency surgery he was uniquely qualified to diagnose his own condition and dictate its management, then again there would have been no problem. He would have been flown to a major institution in Britain or the United States, and would have discussed treatment policy on equal terms with colleagues of equal eminence. As it was, perhaps due to some loss of analytical faculties following the assaults on his brain, he was uncharacteristically indecisive, at times accepting his surgeon's authority (following a lifelong observance of such conventions) but on the other hand attempting to dictate treatment when he disagreed with it. So ended the life of one of the most influential surgeons of the century, a tormented being whose imposing physique concealed a fragile mind, a great teacher unrecognised in his own country, but whose name is still known all over the world. His influence continues, through his writings and through the charitable Trusts which the earnings from those writings have made possible.

CHRONOLOGY

1864	HJB born Forfar
1887	HJB qualifies MB ChB Ed.
1890	HJB marries MB Sent by CMS to Nablus, Palestine Death of their son at two days
1891	Return to UK
1891-95	Medical Directory records Nablus
1894	HHB born Bishopstoke 1 October
1896	Hazelmere, Bishopstoke
1897	At Scotton Road, Bishopstoke
1898	Move to 37 Church Street, Southport May Bailey born
1900	Move to Cavendish Place, Eastbourne
1900	HHB sent to prep school as a boarder (Durley, Southport) principal D. Herridge
1902	Veta Gillender born, daughter of a ship's engineer

1908	Admitted to St Lawrence, Ramsgate From Michaelmas Term 1908 to Summer Term 1910 in Dark Red House (tutor Mr W. Longbourne Smith)
1910	July - won three lengths in school swimming sports Deep sea swimming championship South Coast Summer term, leaves St Lawrence
1911	Takes College of Preceptors Examination, University of Durham
1912	Enters London Hospital Medical College 1 May
1913	OP Dresser 1 July-30 September 'very good'. Gains Honours Certificate in Minor Surgery
1914	May - Approach to Sir Frederick Treves re service in BRC 2 August - Receives telegram from Treves saying 'expedition starts for Belgium tomorrow at 7.30 Charing Cross' Taken prisoner by Germans (Records of British Red Cross record HB as engaged 16 August 1914 and terminated 25 October 1914, *London Hospital Gazette,* December 1914) 23 October - Arrives Newcastle from Belgium via Germany, Denmark, Norway Douro Hoare Prize in Physiology LHMC
1915	Passes 2nd Conjoint Board Fails Primary FRCS Active service with RN (surgeon probationer)
1916	Battle of Jutland. Serves in *Iron Duke*
	<u>Society of Apothecaries</u> Passed surgery 1 January Passed surgery 1 + medicine May Passed forensic medicine and midwifery August (qualified as LMSSA) Gilston Scholarship. LHMC Passed Final Conjt. Medicine and Midwifery August Obstetric student July/August 1916 'good' Medical OP Asst 7 September to 8 October Receiving Room Officer 3 October to 29 October House Surgeon to Rigby and Milne 30 Oct to 5 Jan

1917	Passed Final Conjoint Surgery January (MRCS LRCP) (Diploma awarded 8 February) Promoted to Surg Lt RN June 1917 - Served on M19 in Mediterranean Posted as MO to German Navy off Scapa Flow
1918	Tansferred to Portsmouth, then to Granton Hospital, Edinburgh
1919	Discharged from RN
1920	Final FRCS - 15 September 25 October - Recorded as passing 'operative surgery'. FRCS diploma November Address in Medical Directory as 100 Rugby Rd Brighton (temp. Surg. Lt RN) House surgeon LH
1921	18 January - Appointed RSO, General Hospital Wolverhampton 27 June Unsuccessful application to LH as registrar June - Appointed surgical registrar at Liverpool RI October - Admitted as 'country member' of Liverpool Medical Institution
1922	6 February - Appointed as Surgical Registrar at LH. Worked as SR from 27 February 1922 to 30 March 1923 March - Returned to London Title of post changed to First Assistant in October 1923. Became Clinical Assistant to G.U. Department
1923	1 October 1923 to 28 February 1925 - 1st Asst to Sir H. Rigby and Mr J. Walton Address 12 Brunswick Road, Hove 15 February 1923 - Appointed as Surgical Registrar at LH
1924	Continued in post as First Assistant Loss of left index finger
1925	Unsuccessful application for post as Consultant Surgeon to the London Hospital

	Appointed Honorary Assistant Surgeon to Liverpool Royal Infirmary Gillson Scholarship, Society of Apothecaries Meets Veta Gillender who was working in a photographic studio (address given as 65 Blandford St W1) July - Appointed to Dudley Road Hospital Birmingham (address 32 Wheatsheaf Road, near Edgbaston Reservoir)
1926	14 January - Marries Veta 1st edition of *PSCS* produced at DRH Started work on ES
1927	1st edition of *PSCS* appears
1928	at DRH
1929	Appointed to Bruce Wills Memorial Hospital Bristol (later Bristol Homeopathic) Fails to be appointed to BRI 1st edition *ES* appears
1930	25 November - Appointed to staff of RNH at the same time as RMcNL JHB buys the house in Hendon
1931	First operation at RNH (Ca pinna) 27 January - First attendance at Medical Ctee at RNH
1932	Moves to Mill Hill (Mote Ho, Courtland Ave, London NW7) Starts work at Oldchurch 1st edition of *Bailey & Love SPS* Veta's second pregnancy terminated at March (hyperemesis)
1933	Entry in Medical Directory reads HJB 'recently deceased' (died in surgery from embolus while sitting in chair having seen patients) (address 123 Harley St, London)
1934	Moves to Fairlawn
1935	Starts work at Clacton Appointed as Executive Treasurer Europe for ICS
1940	1st edition of *Surgery of Modern Warfare* appears

	RNH receives direct hit Zina Fitzgerald (nee Moncrieff) HS at RNH Later OPMO and Cas Officer. Not HB's HS but knew of his work
1943	29 July - Death on train of Hamilton junior returning from St Bees. ICS Conference 18 December - HB receives diploma on behalf of RMcNL in NY
1944	1st edition of *Notable Names*, with W. J. Bishop
1945	RCS bombed. ICS sent $2000 to help in reconstruction. Cheque received by HB who sent 'lovely letter of acknowlegement'
1946	24 March - ICS meets in Lima. HB present by proxy AC appointed to RNH as HS to HB and WBG
1947	Hunterian Professorial Lecture at Royal College of Surgeons on 'Parotidectomy' Applies for Chair of Surgery in Cape Town on retirement of Charles Saint ICS Chicago Last operation at RNH 4 April - recommends Zachary Cope for FICS
1948	ICS Rome. Recorded as attending in person Proposed as President, but withdrew his nomination in favour of Dr Herbert Acuff Last recorded attendance at RNH Medical Ctee
1949	27 April - RNH Medical Cttee receives letter from HB announcing his resignation
1949-50	In hospital ICS New York
1950	25 April RNH Medical Ctee decides that HB should not be replaced by urologist
1951	Admitted to Graylingwell Hospital Chichester Receives ECT Leucotomy suggested but refused by Veta

	Receives Lithium
	Sister May dies (?at 53)
1954	29 January - HB discharged from Graylingwell 5 February - HB and VB fly to Tenerife 3 May - Living in Cornwall. Relapse. Letter from Dr Eddison to G'well
1956	Hull Place, Sholden nr Deal 31 December - letter from Mr Bowesma Kumasi Central Hospital
1959	Hawkinge, nr Folkestone 25 December - letter re review of *Basic Surgery* writen by John Bruce
1960	Moves to Fuengirola
1961	26 March - Death of HHB in Malaga
1962	Veta builds Los Arcos
1989	Death of Veta

BIBLIOGRAPHY

ARTICLES BY HAMILTON BAILEY

(not including chapters in books edited by other authors)

With the British Red Cross in Belgium	*London Hosp Gazette* Dec. 1914
Clinical aspects of branchial cysts	*Br J Surg* 1922 10: 565
Injuries of kidneys and ureter	*Br J Surg* 1924 11: 609
Submaxillary salivary calculi	*Br J Surg* 1924 11: 807
Excision of the ureter (with G. Huddy)	*Br J Surg* 1924 11: 943
Studies in the male breast	*Lancet* 1924 1: 1258
An unbreakable suture needle	*Br J Surg* 1924
Thyroglosal cysts and fistulae	*Br J Surg* 1925 12: 579
True congenital thyroglossal fistulae	*Proc Roy Soc Med* 1925 18: 6
Abdominal crises in pernicious anaemia	*Br Med J* 1926 2: 554
Spinal anaesthesia in intussusception	*Lancet* 1926 2: 648
Clinical aspects of acute pancreatitis	*Br Med J* 1926 1: 367
The value of Loewi's test in acute pancreatitis	*Practitioner* 1926 117: 122
Hydrocele of femoral hernial sac	*Br J Surg* 1927 15: 166
Screwdriver for ox-bone plates	*Lancet* 1927 2: 396
Bone grafts in Pott's disease	*Birm Med Rev* 1927 2: 331
Notes on drainage of pelvic abscess	*Lancet* 1927 2: 754
Traumatic rupture of the normal spleen	*Br J Surg* 1927
Testicular grafting	*Lancet* 1927 1: 1284
Impending death under anaesthesia	*Practitioner* 1927 118: 368
Branchial fistula	*Clin J* 1927 56: 619
Rupture of the urethra	*Br J Surg* 1928 15: 370
Traction fracture of the small trochanter	*J Bone Joint Surg* 1928 10: 336
Ligation of the angular vein in facial carbuncle	*Surg Gynec Obstet* 1928 46: 565
Raynaud's disease treated by sympathectomy	*Br J Surg* 1928 16: 160
Diagnosis of branchial cyst	*Br Med J* 1928 1: 940
Volkmann's ischaemic contracture	*Br J Surg* 1928 16: 335
Notes on strangulated incisional hernia	*Lancet* 1928 2: 812

Probe pointed scissors for salivary calculi	*Lancet* 1928 2: 232
Strangulated femoral hernia	*Br Med J* 1928 2: 1033
Nephro-ureteral anastomosis	*J Urol* 1928 20:, 103
Meralgia paraesthetica	*Clin J* 1928 57: 391
Acute intussusception in adults	*Birm Med Rev* 1928 3: 287
Physical signs in acute abdominal catastrophes	*M Rev of Med* 1929 35
Ochsner-Sherren treatment of acute appendicitis	*Br Med J* 1929 1: 140
Aspirating the contents of the stomach	*Br Med J* 1929 2: 854
Suppurating deep iliac glands	*Practitioner* 1929 124: 223
Use of ox bone plates in fractures	*Lancet* 1929 1: 820
Diaphysectomy in osteomyelitis	*Br Med J* 1930 17: 64
Adenitis of facial lymph nodes	*Practitioner* 1930 125: 618
Facio-cervical actinomycosis	*Postgrad Med J* 1930 6: 128
Spontaneous rupture of the normal spleen	*Br J Surg* 1930 17: 417
Purpura as an acute abdominal emergency	*Br J Surg* 1930 18: 234
Haemangioma of kidney	*Br J Urol* 1930 2: 375
Alarming rectal haemorrhage in typhoid	*Lancet* 1931 1: 1294
Stones in the submaxillary gland	*Practitioner* 1931 126: 671
Ranula	*Br Dent J* 1931 52: 581
Complete eradication of the thyroglossal tract	*Br Med J* 1931 2: 13
Ludwig's angina	*Practitioner* 1931 127: 365
Tuberculous cervical adenitis	*Clin J* 1931 60: 409
Tuberculous cervical abscess and branchial cyst	*Br J Tuberc* 1931 25
Surgical emergencies of kidney	*Practitioner* 1933 130: 342
Treatment of bladder paralysis	*Practitioner* 1933 130: 347
Treatment of abscess of the breast	*Br Med J* 1933 1: 1001
Maldescent of the testis	*Postgrad Med J* 1933 4: 247
Clinical aspects of branchial fistula	*Br J Surg* 1933 21: 173
Apparatus for local anaesthesia	*Lancet* 1933 2: 922
Continuous intravenous saline *(with J. M. Carnow)*	*Br Med J* 1934 1: 11
Salivary glands	*Practitioner* 1934 132: 151
Decompression of the bladder	*Br J Urol* 1934 6: 225
Some recent advances in surgery	*Practitioner* 1935 135: 526
Addison's disease treated by adrenal grafting *(with K. D. Keele)*	*Proc Roy Soc Med* 1935 29: 42
A tube for continuous gastric aspiration	*Lancet* 1936 1: 150
A pocket transilluminator	*Lancet* 1936 1: 906
Plastic operations for hydronephrosis	*Br Med J* 1936 2: 669
Perforated peptic ulcer	*Lancet* 1936 2: 249
Cystic hygroma	*Clin J* 1937 66: 242
Continuous intravenous saline infusions *(with W. I. B. Stringer , K. D. Keele)*	*Br Med J* 1937 1: 152
Interception and regulation of intravenous saline	*Lancet* 1937 2: 24
Transverse upper abdominal incisions	*Trans Int Coll Surg* 1938
Reconstruction of the deep urethra	*Br J Urol* 1939 11: 111
Sublingual dermoids	*Br J Surg* 1939 27: 140
A syringe for sialography	*Lancet* 1939 2: 80
Cystic hygroma	*J Int Coll Surg* 1939
Excision of the total leukoplakic area of the tongue	*J Int Coll Surg* 1939
Median mental sinus	*Br Dental J* 1939

Leontiasis Ossia	*Br Dental J* 1939
Incontinence of urine treated by a gracilis sling	*Br J Urol* 1939 11: 280
Two cases of complete removal of the parotid gland	*Proc Roy Soc Med* 1939 32: 138
Addison's disease treated by adrenal graft (*with K. D. Keele*)	*Proc Roy Soc Med* 1939 32: 384
Electrosurgical obliteration of the gallbladder (*with R. J. M. Love*)	*Br Med J* 1939 2: 682
Ether convulsions	*Br Med J* 1940 2: 222
Inflammation of the tongue	*Clin J* 1940 69: 253
Drug after treatment for infected hands	*Lancet* 1941 2: 189
Treatment of tumours of the parotid gland	*Br J Surg* 1941 28 337
Cardiac massage for impending death	*Br Med J* 1941 2: 84
Open surgical treatment of tuberculous abscesses	*J Int Coll Surg* 1942 5: 275
Persistent hiccup	*Practitioner* 1942 150: 173
Gas gangrene (*with R. J. McNeill Love*)	*J Int Coll Surg* 1943 6: 275
Bone marrow as a site for infusion	*Br Med J* 1944 1: 181
Blast injury	*J Int Coll Surg* 1944 7: 257
Crush Syndrome	*J Int Coll Surg* 1944 7: 343
Congenital parotid sialectasis	*J Int Coll Surg* 1945 8: 109
Local infiltration of procaine	*J Int Coll Surg* 1945 8: 427
Obstructive anuria	*Br J Urol* 1945 17: 118
Treatment of collar-stud abscess	*Br J Surg* 1945 33: 53
Differential diagnosis of renal colic	*Urol Cutan Rev* 1946 50: 398
Impending death under anesthesia	*Lancet* 1947 1: 5
Impending death under anesthesia	*J Int Coll Surg* 1947 10: 1
Some clinical entities frequently misdiagnosed	*J Int Coll Surg* 1947
Parotidectomy: indications and results	*Br Med J* 1947 1: 404
Sternal trocar and cannula	*Br Med J* 1947 1: 459
Discontinuous intravenous infusions	*Br Med J* 1947 2: 333
Ectopic gestation	*Clin Med* 1947 57: 347
Tuberculous cervical adenitis	*Lancet* 1948 1: 313
Persistent priapism	*Br J Surg* 1948 35: 298
Subphrenic abscess	*J Int Coll Surg* 1948 11: 207
The National Health Service	*J Int Coll Surg* 1948
Phlebothrombosis and pulmonary embolus	*Br Med J* 1948 1: 594
Surgical anatomy of the parotid gland	*Br Med J* 1948 2: 245
Differential diagnosis of tuberculous adenitis	*Tubercle* 1948 29: 174
Parotidectomía	*Semana Medica* 1949 1: 558
The technique of parotidectomy	*J Int Coll Surg* 1949 12: 103
Air embolism	*J Int Coll Surg* 1956 25: 675
Infections of the foot	*J IntColl Surg* 1957 27:475
Oxygen therapy	*J Int Coll Surg* 1957 28: 519
Gram's stain	*J Int Coll Surg* 1959 31: 10
Reiter's disease	*Br J Ven Dis* 1959 35: 101
Reiter's disease	*J Int Coll Surg* 1960 33: 17
The cradle of blood transfusion in Britain	*J Int Coll Surg* 1961 35: 28

BOOKS BY HAMILTON BAILEY

Demonstrations of Physical Signs in Clinical Surgery
First edition: Bristol, John Wright, 1927
Subsequent editions 1930, 1931, 1933, 1935, 1937, 1940, 1942, 1944, 1946, 1949, 1954, 1957
By Allan Clain: 1960 1967, 1973, 1977, 1986
By John Lumley 1997

German edition 1939, 1956, 1959
Turkish edition 1943
Spanish edition 1947
Hungarian edition 1948
Yugoslav edition 1953
Chinese edition 1956

Branchial Cysts and Other Conditions in the Cervico-Facial Region.
London, H. K. Lewis, 1929

Emergency Surgery
First edition: Bristol, John Wright 1930
Subsequent editions 1933, 1936, 1938, 1940, 1944, 1953, 1958
By T. J. McNair: 1967, 1972,
By H. A. F. Dudley: 1977,1986
By B. W. Ellis and S. Paterson-Brown: 1995

A Short Practice of Surgery (with R. J. McNeill Love)
First edition: London, H. K. Lewis 1932
Subsequent editions 1935, 1936, 1938, 1941, 1946, 1948, 1952, 1956, 1959
With J. Charnley: 1962
By A. J. H. Rains and J Charnley 1965
By A. J. H. Rains and W M Capper 1968, 1971
By A. J. H. Rains & D Ritchie: 1975, 1981
By A. J. H. Rains & C V Mann: 1984, 1988
By C. V. Mann & R C G Russell: 1992
By C. V. Mann, R C G Russell & N L Williams: 1995

Surgery for Nurses (with R. J. McNeill Love)
First edition: London, H. K. Lewis 1933
Subsequent editions: 1936, 1940, 1945, 1948, 1950, 1954

Diseases of the Testicle. London, H. K. Lewis, 1936

Clinical Surgery for Dental Practitioners.
First edition: London, H. K. Lewis, 1936
Second edition, 1937

Recent Advances in Genitourinary Surgery (with N. M. Matheson).
Edinburgh, Churchill Livingstone, 1936

Pye's Surgical Handicraft
Eleventh edition: 1938
Subsequent editions: 1940, 1944
With Alan Kark: 1947
By Allan Clain: 1956, 1962

The Surgery of Modern Warfare
First edition: Edinburgh, Churchill Livingston, 1940
Subsequent editions: 1942, 1944

Notable Names in Medicine and Surgery (with W. J. Bishop)
First edition: London, H. K. Lewis, 1944
Subsequent editions: 1946, 1959
By H. Ellis: 1983

101 Clinical Demonstrations for Nurses
First edition: Edinburgh, Churchill Livingstone, 1944
Subsequent editions: 1946, 1954
Revised by A. R. Isaac: 1961, 1967

Unfinished

Surgery of the Neck

Surgical Diagnosis

INDEX

A

B

C

D

E

F

G

H

I

J

K

L

M

N

O

P

R

S

T

U

V

W

For EU product safety concerns, contact us at Calle de José Abascal, 56–1°, 28003 Madrid, Spain or eugpsr@cambridge.org.

www.ingramcontent.com/pod-product-compliance
Lightning Source LLC
LaVergne TN
LVHW011804200926
848484LV00003B/781